Walking
the Walk

Walking the Walk

∾ Getting Fit with Faith ∾

Leslie Sansone
with Rowan Jacobsen

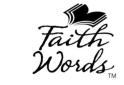

NEW YORK BOSTON NASHVILLE

Scriptures are taken from the *Holy Bible: New International Version*®. Copyright © 1973, 1978, 1984 by International Bible Society. Used by permission of Zondervan Publishing House. All rights reserved.

FaithWords

Hachette Book Group USA
237 Park Avenue, New York, NY 10017
Visit our Web site at www.faithwords.com

The FaithWords name and logo are registered trademarks of the Hachette Book Group USA
Printed in the United States of America

First edition: July 2007

10   9   8   7   6   5   4   3   2   1

Library of Congress Cataloging-in-Publication Data
Sansone, Leslie.
    Walking the walk : getting fit with faith / Leslie Sansone with Rowan Jacobsen. — 1st ed.
       p.   cm.
ISBN: 978-0-446-58104-2
1. Fitness walking—Religious aspects—Christianity.   2. Physical fitness—Religious aspects—Christianity.   3. Walking—Religious aspects—Christianity.   I. Jacobsen, Rowan.   II. Title.
RA78.65.S233   2007
613.7'176—dc22
                                                                        2006038186

Contents

Walking
the Walk

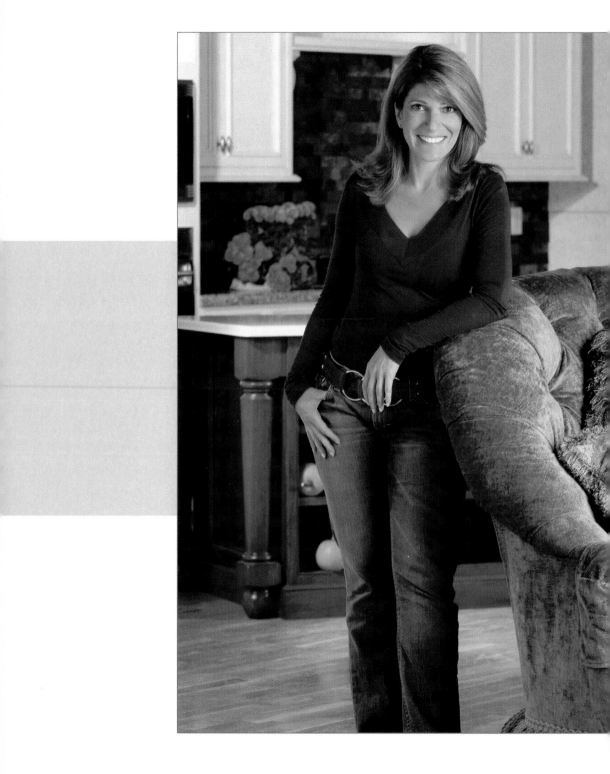

Introduction

The power of faith is awesome. Look around you, and you'll know this to be true. Faith built the great cathedrals of Europe and America. Faith built the towns, structure, and social fabric of this frontier nation. Faith really *has* moved mountains. Faith drives the success of some of our greatest humanitarians, businesspeople, and athletes.

Look inside yourself, and you'll know this to be true even more. For most of us, faith goes hand in hand with success, happiness, and peace. This isn't a coincidence. When you are aware of the deeper reasons why you do something, aware that you are part of something much bigger than yourself, you are much more likely to stick to it. The reverse is true, too. When your faith wavers, it can be hard to see the point in doing anything.

That's why I believe that the single best way to get fit is with faith. You may not be able to find the willpower to make yourself walk every day, but if you turn around and ask God to help you out of bed and into your sneakers, it will work almost every time. My faith has walked me through disappointment, heartache, anger, stress . . . all the normal emotions we experience in life.

You may think you are so out of shape that only a miracle could get you exercising, but miracles happen every day. And as miracles go, your getting in shape is a pretty small one. In the Bible, of course, there is the story of the crippled man whose friends took him to see Jesus. The room Jesus was in was so crowded, they couldn't even get their lame friend inside, so they climbed onto the roof and lowered him in from there on his mat. Jesus said to the man, "Rise, take up thy bed, and walk." And to the astonishment of everybody, the man did.

You are no cripple, but with the help of this book, and your faith, you, too, are going to rise from the couch, take up thy DVD, and walk! As I said, in the range of miracles, this is small potatoes. But the change in how you'll look and feel will seem miraculous to you.

Think about Lazarus. He was dead four days by the time Jesus arrived at his tomb. Yet Jesus was able to make Lazarus rise from the dead. Now, you may *feel* like death warmed over, and you may be in a dark place where you don't believe you'll ever be able to achieve anything again, much less get in shape, but you are doing *way* better than Lazarus! The only things you need to rise again and regain your energy, health, and happiness are a little faith and a little support—and in this book, I'm here to provide the first steps of that support.

But I can't do it alone. For this to work, your commitment is required. I'll give you the plan for achieving health and fitness, and you'll pony up the dedication to really give it a try and to truly open yourself to letting God take charge. I call it "energetic worship." If you and I do our part, God will do the rest.

I wrote this book to encourage you to be a lifelong believer! A believer that healthy choices really do make this journey of life better. A believer that faith is a major component of healthy living. A believer that *you* have everything it takes to get everything you want in life. Are you ready to believe? Because I am ready to believe in you.

⌣ Why Faith? ⌣

This is about achieving wholeness. If you are physically healthy, well rested, and feeling grounded in your life, if your purpose is clear and your mental stamina is sharp, it will be easy to move forward.

The flip side is that when one piece of your life gets out of whack, it can throw the rest off, too. That's how a lot of us get out of shape to begin with. We certainly never intend to start eating poorly or to be inactive, but it creeps up on us. Maybe you took a job that involved long hours at a desk; when you got off work, you barely had time to grab some unhealthy take-out food and collapse, exhausted, in front of the tube for a couple of hours before falling asleep and doing the whole thing over again the next day. Or maybe you suffered an injury or arthritis in a knee, which kept you off your feet and forced you to abandon your exercise program. Soon you gained weight and found it even harder to stay active. And this, of course, took a toll on your spirit. The more out of shape you got, the more down you became, and the less you could see any point in trying to turn the tide.

Over the past thirty years, I've worked with thousands of women who, for one reason or another, found themselves caught in traps like this. Their lives got out of balance, exercise was the first casualty, and often they took solace in food because of their bruised self-image. It's a vicious cycle. But what I've heard from so many of these women—and know to be true myself—is that the key to escaping this cycle is *faith*.

The spiritual part of ourselves is the strongest and the most sensitive at the same time. It can show incredible resiliency and force in the most trying of circumstances, but it's also the part most easily obscured by day-to-day life. Or maybe the quiet murmurings of the spirit can't compete with the thunderous demands of bosses, kids, stomachs, and bank accounts. But re-acquainting yourself with spirit is the way to bring wholeness back into your life—and regaining that wholeness is going to be your focus for the next thirty days. It's about getting healthy, body and soul, but, as I like to say, the goal is less body, more soul!

❧ How It Works ❧

This book is designed to help you harness the power of faith—whatever your personal faith may be—and use it to help you finally achieve your desire to lose weight, get fit, shake off health problems, and find success and meaning in *every* day. Each day for the next thirty days, you and I will focus on a different piece of the faith/fitness puzzle, using spirituality to support your quest to get physically healthy, and, in return, using the great energy and contentment generated by physical activity to reaffirm your spiritual commitment. We might spend one day considering how prayer or meditation can strengthen your resolve to stick to your weight-loss goals, and another day recognizing that food is sacred and that how we think of it influences how we eat.

No matter what the day's topic, you'll be walking with me, using the DVD provided with this book. You can go at whatever pace works for you.

You can start at a gentle half mile and work your way up, or start with a mile, or do the full three miles from the get-go. The important thing for long-term success is to do it almost every day, and that can be achieved by keeping things at the "doable challenge" level, where you actually look forward to them.

Each day of the program includes reminders to meet your exercise goals, as well as space for tracking your progress. Another section gives you an inspiring scriptural quote to get your day off on the right note, along with some questions for deeper reflection on the day's topic. Affirmations help you keep walking through doubt, and activities are suggested that can help you improve your health, cultivate your faith, and help others to do the same. Fit Facts are provided to help you understand why simple changes in behavior can greatly impact your looks, health, and mind-set. Nobody likes to be burdened with page after page of boring information on nutrition and health, so I've made it easy on you by providing just three amazing bite-size facts to take in each day. You'll love quoting them to your friends and helping them get on track, too. If they need more convincing, they can read the testimonies (A Witness for Fitness) from individuals who have used my program and their faith to change their lives and those of others. These walking wonders will convince anyone that it really works!

Now, you may be so hungry to achieve permanent weight loss that you're thinking, Leslie, I don't want to lose weight steadily and gradually; I want to walk off some serious pounds as fast as I can, and I'm willing to do what it takes! If that's the case, then have I got just the plan for you! Flip to the appendix and get started right away on my 7-Day "Jump Start" Weight-Loss Plan. It demands a lot of eating discipline from you, but it will also blast your calorie burn not just through the roof but into the stratosphere! To prepare yourself for that journey, you will need all three kinds of fuel that this book provides:

1. Fuel for the mind: Read the day's chapter in this book for inspiration and focus.
2. Fuel for the body: Eat healthy, energizing foods, such as those listed in the weekly meal plan in the appendix.

3. Fuel for the spirit: Walk all three miles with me on the enclosed DVD to burn calories and uplift your emotions and spirit.

That's it! Simple, huh? But oh so effective.

But remember: Nothing is required of you in this book. Everything is here for your benefit. There are no tests or assignments. You get to pick and choose what helps you and what you want to ignore. Even if you just use this book for inspiration, it will pay off by improving your quality of life. If you just walk with the DVD, you will be walking off pounds. If you just read the Fit Facts, you will start making smart health choices. If you do it all, you will be so joyful and proud. But it's your choice. You need to walk *your* walk in life; I hope that with this book I can help you do that.

ᵔ What Faith Means to Me ᵔ

I know what a difference faith has made in my own life. I started teaching aerobics in the 1980s, after I discovered how incredible working out made me feel. Sure, I felt healthier, lost weight, and toned my body, giving me much better self-esteem. But I also turbocharged my energy level. Most important of all, I turbocharged my spirit! A half hour of aerobic exercise and I felt like somebody had shaken the dust off an antenna and plugged it into my spiritual receiver. I could feel Spirit working through me, and wanted as many others as possible to experience this same joy.

I started off my career by teaching aerobics in church basements. I didn't charge a fee; I just set out a coffee can for donations. Thinking back on it now, it seems perfect to me that it all started in church basements. It was my calling, after all: the best way for me to fulfill my Christian commitment to serve God by serving others. I found the people who were looking for what I offered through church networks, and it all snowballed from there. Today, I reach a lot more people through TV and videos than I did going from church to church, but it's still true that a lot of what binds us together is our belief in the goodness of what we do, and the foundation for that is our relationship with God.

For me, that relationship has existed since I was a child. As with all truly loving relationships, it is one that keeps getting stronger and more rewarding every year. I grew up in a Pennsylvania Italian-American Catholic family. Like many such families, we dutifully went to church and followed all the Catholic traditions, but our faith didn't involve much inner commitment.

The first big influence that made me realize faith could go much deeper than that was my older sister, Toni. I remember her as a teenager, reading the Bible on her bed. I started getting more involved, too, but then in my twenties, I started to experiment. It's a natural, healthy process for children to grow, test their faith, question things, and then of their own accord fall into deep belief. I never wavered from Christianity, but I did explore a number of different churches. I loved the pure energy you could get from a Baptist or evangelical service. I was open to all denominations. I would go wherever good things were being preached!

What turned me off about some experiences was when a service felt canned—anytime it didn't feed my soul. Worse still was when I heard Jesus' lessons being used not to bring positive change but, instead, to judge others. Over time, I found the churches that resonated with my own beliefs and needs. And with every year, I understand more and more the incredible opportunity being granted to us through His love.

I wouldn't say that there was one single moment where lightning struck and set me on my current path, but I have had several experiences where I suddenly felt God's love shining powerfully within me, which helped me commit even more strongly to my path. The one I recall most vividly was in New Orleans, many years ago, at the end of a four-day convention. After visiting Bourbon Street the night before and seeing some of the desperate extremes people will go to in the name of "fun," I was feeling a little down. There was a gorgeous Catholic church on the square near where I was staying, so I decided to attend the Sunday-morning service before catching my plane.

Churches are my favorite buildings on this earth. I love the look of a church, the smell of a church, the sounds of a church. When I am in a church, I am deeply connected to God with all my senses. And this church was no exception. The priest there gave the most powerful sermon I've ever heard! His message was on living Jesus' teachings in your daily life, all the time, not just for a couple of hours a week. The squalor of Bourbon Street the night before made his message all the more poignant.

As I was leaving the church after the service, the priest was in the back. Our eyes met. We both had tears in them. At that moment, I felt how incredibly good God is to us, and reaffirmed my commitment to further His work in everything I do.

I think my faith expresses itself in many ways—not all of them traditional ones. It's part of my commitment to getting as many people as possible fit and healthy so they can lead active, loving lives. It shows in my membership in several different churches and ministries. I hope it shows in my caring treatment of other people. Perhaps most of all, it is a part of my commitment to raising my kids in as loving an environment as possible. Knowing that they have God's love, as well as my own, helps give them the inner security they need to grow up to be positive, loving adults.

In a world that seems to be filled with so much anger, danger, and misunderstanding, I believe it is more important than ever to try to live in the Light at all times. For me, that means Walking the Walk every day. I believe that the Word of God is absolute, and that He will take us to a higher level every time. Keeping this in mind helps me to strive for that higher level in everything I do. And I don't take any of this for granted—I've been incredibly blessed to have this influence in my life; it's my ultimate good fortune.

Arise and Walk!

Over the next thirty days, you're going to be doing some good hard thinking about your life, your body, and your goals. But today is not one of those days! It's easy to overthink a situation. You can think about a problem so much that you bury yourself in the thinking and never get around to doing anything about it. Sometimes it's necessary to *just do it*! A lot of things that seemed confusing or insurmountable become clear once you're actively making progress.

Today is your *just do it* day.

Plan a time when you can sneak in a half hour to walk with me. If you haven't exercised in a long time, then fifteen minutes is fine. The important thing is that you actually do it. Once you've got one day under your belt and see how easy and fun it is, the rest of the days will be a piece of cake.

Part of this has to do with breaking your patterns. We sometimes think of our spirit, body, and mind as three separate things, but they are intimately connected. Any change in one affects the others. Mental stress shows up in our face, skin, and graying hair, and can even cause us to gain weight. A sagging spirit can easily take down our bodies with it. But the flip side is true, too. We've had the experience of feeling sluggish or depressed and of thinking we just want to sleep, but then we do something active, like take a walk or go for a swim, and our entire outlook changes. Suddenly, we have tons of energy and the future looks a whole lot better! We managed to revive our mind and spirit through the body!

Call this "runner's high." Call it "walking away the blues." Call it whatever you want. Just know that it works. You can change your patterns and change your life. A daily walk is a perfect place to start to make this come true.

That's why if you're down in the dumps about your weight or health, the worst thing to do is overanalyze it. Get up and walk instead! Not only will you actually make an impact on your weight and health but you'll raise your spirits more than any amount of mental gymnastics ever could.

∿ Having Faith ∿

See if you recognize yourself in any of these un-faith-full thought patterns. Today, try to switch your inner dialogue so that your mind walks the walk along with your body.

Un-Faith-Full Thoughts:

- I always fail weight-loss programs. I was meant to be overweight.
- Exercise is harder for me than it is for other people. Why even try?
- I'm just getting older. It's a losing battle. If I'd started in my twenties, I'd still have time to get fit.

Walking the Walk:

"Today is today. By walking with spirit, I'll make it a great day. And tomorrow will be even better."

∿ Walking for Other Reasons ∿

"Whoever claims to live in him must walk as Jesus did."
1 JOHN 2:6

I like to think that I walk with God in all that I do, but I really feel it when I'm walking. Walking is a form of energetic worship, just like singing in a Baptist church. It's also something Jesus did a great deal in His lifetime. Walking has a strong Christian tradition.

True, the Bible doesn't make a big deal about walking for exercise—or about any other form of exercise, for that matter. Does that mean people didn't need exercise back then? Of course not. People walked *every day.* They had no choice. No one needed to worry about getting exercise to improve their health or lose weight; physical activity was a given. What they needed to worry about was consuming enough calories to supply their needs! With no cars or public transportation, almost all travel in the early Christian era was on foot.

In His lifetime, Jesus walked thousands and thousands of miles. As a child, He most likely traveled from Nazareth to Jerusalem many times. In the course of His ministry, He traveled from Galilee to Jerusalem, into the wilderness and back, and throughout Israel. He probably walked many miles most days. While this would make Him a champion walker in our era, He thought nothing of this, and it's likely that His contemporaries didn't, either: They were walking nearly as much! The apostle Paul traveled many thousands of miles on his missionary journeys to Greece and beyond.

Would Paul have taken a car or train if he'd had the opportunity? Certainly. And it wouldn't have been practical for Jesus to walk throughout Israel if everyone else had been zipping around in Toyotas. But He *did* walk, and it must have helped energize Him, too. When I walk, I like to remember that I'm engaging in an activity that directly connects me to a two-thousand-year-old tradition of inspired walkers serving the Lord by putting one foot in front of the other. Just look at how many times the Bible uses walking as a metaphor for the spiritual path, from "And walk in love, as Christ also has loved us" to "We walk by faith, not by sight."

When *you* walk, know that you aren't doing it just for yourself. Taking the time to care for your body is a direct path to physical, mental, and *spiritual* fitness. Above all things, it is your spiritual fitness that will lead to a successful life on this planet and will help you further God's plan.

∿ Activities ∿

On the future days of this thirty-day program, I'll suggest various activities you can do to start working that day's topic into your life. But on this first day, I don't want you to worry about anything but walking. I have just one activity to suggest for today, and it is a *non*activity.

Turn off the analysis machine in your head. Today, don't criticize yourself, don't compliment yourself, and don't evaluate your performance in any way. Just do. The more you think things to death, the less likely you will be to act. This is your day to act instinctively and unhesitatingly—in everything you do, but especially in beginning your walking program.

Fit Facts

The Nitric-Oxide Breakthrough

Steady cardiovascular exercise, such as walking, running, or cycling, causes your body to release nitric oxide throughout your cells. This chemical helps dilate blood vessels and increase blood flow throughout the body, allowing extra energy and oxygen to reach your muscles when you need them, but it also increases the flow of neurochemicals in your brain. You think faster and more creatively. So yes, walking literally changes the way you think about things!

Endorphins to the Rescue

Cardiovascular exercise also causes the release in the brain of endorphins—natural "feel good" chemicals. That's why you feel so good after exercise. Several studies have found that regular exercise is as effective as antidepressants in treating mild depression—and it sometimes works in cases where antidepressants don't. Perhaps the best long-term mental impact of exercise is the self-esteem it gives you, knowing that you've improved your looks and health along with your outlook. That's an effect drugs can't match!

Walk Away Those Pounds

You burn about two hundred calories doing the two-mile walk as demonstrated on the enclosed DVD. Do that most days each week and you'll burn away twenty pounds of fat in a year. Your change in dress size will be even more dramatic, because all that walking uses up fat and builds lean, sleek muscle, giving you the tone you want.

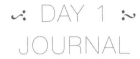

⌐ DAY 1 ⌐
JOURNAL
Arise and Walk!

Affirmation

"The strength I need to get fit is already inside me.
Starting today, I will call on that strength every day,
and I know it will guide me."

Today's Walk

How Far? _____

Strength Training? _____

How'd It Go? _____

Notes

_____

_____

_____

Walking on Purpose

"Did you do that on purpose?" a friend might ask when you decide to stand up on a bus just as someone else is looking for a seat. What she wants to know is if there was intent behind your action. But I'd like to think that, in an ideal life, there is intent behind *all* our actions. Everything we do should be "on purpose."

We all sometimes wonder about our purpose in life. But we can get bogged down by confusing our purpose with our job or hobbies or standing in the community. Your purpose isn't a thing; it isn't how you describe yourself in a mortgage application; it's the action you take every day and the reverence you feel while doing it.

One of the best ways of telling if you are doing something on purpose is whether, while you're doing it, you are asking yourself, Is this part of my purpose? Asking that question would be a sure sign that you were *off* purpose. Beethoven didn't worry about his purpose in life while he was writing his symphonies; he just wrote. Mother Teresa didn't worry about her purpose; she just fed the poor.

We tend to think of life purposes as serving big altruistic causes—caring for the poor or saving endangered species, for example—but all God asks from us is right living; doing what's right, serving others, modeling a healthy life for the next generation. Simply knowing that we are acting out of integrity and love is far more important than getting hung up on the outcome of our quest.

You may ask, "How can something as mundane as walking be part of my purpose in life?" For one answer to that question, read today's "Walking for Other Reasons." For another, think about how good walking makes you feel—not just after the activity but during it, too. If halfway through a walk, you are completely into it, moving in step with the rhythm and music and not thinking about anything else at all, then you can rest assured that you are on purpose. Being deeply engaged in life at that basic level *is* the point.

One of the main reasons people shirk exercise is because they feel it isn't part of their purpose. They know it's good for them, but if it is taking time away from what they see as their purpose—and let's face it, exercise does take time—then their hearts and souls won't be in it. Starting today, on Day 2 of your recommitment to yourself, try to make that mental shift to accepting physical activity as part of your purpose. It isn't wasted time; it's devotional time. Embrace it to the point that you don't even think about it. Make it so that when you finish a walk, if somebody were to stop by and ask, "Did you do that on purpose?" you would raise your chin high and say, "Yep, I sure did."

◡ Having Faith ◡

See if you recognize yourself in any of these un-faith-full thought patterns. Today, try to switch your inner dialogue so that your mind walks the walk along with your body.

Un-Faith-Full Thoughts:

- ↬ I'm wasting my life. I should have lived it differently.
- ↬ I don't need good health. I'd rather concentrate on others.
- ↬ Why should my life have meaning? I'm not important enough.

Walking the Walk:

"My body is my temple. When I honor my body, I honor God."

✌ Walking for Other Reasons ✌

". . . let us not love with words or tongue
but with actions and in truth."

I JOHN 3:18

Why do you want to get fit? The women who come to my classes at Studio Fitness or do my videos have a fantastic variety of reasons for wanting to get fit, but a few are perennial favorites. One is health. They might have received a wake-up call from their doctor: If they want to be around in ten years without debilitating conditions like diabetes, they'd better start moving. Many women have young children and commit to a healthier lifestyle for the sake of their kids. Some are just tired of the limitations that come with being overweight: physical limitations, limitations on what you can wear, and social limitations that come with the stigma of being overweight in America.

Of course, being overweight is a human concept. So is being thin, or attractive, or old. These all have to do with comparing yourself to other people. And God doesn't care about any of that. So does God care if you're fit?

I believe so, but not for the reasons you might think.

Go back to the reasons most women start walking with me. They want to lose weight and look better, yes—so that they can do whatever they want physically without being out of breath, so that they can feel confident about themselves, and so that they can spend many years with their loved ones without having health conditions that confine them. For these women, getting fit is about removing self-imposed limitations.

You could say that our main goal in life is to remove limitations. Sometimes we get stuck focusing on worldly limitations: We want more money to be able to buy whatever we desire, a more powerful job that allows us to make more decisions, convenience stores and fast-food restaurants that don't limit our time, and so on. But ultimately what we're after in life is removing any limitations from our relationship with God. We want to be one with Spirit and enjoy the infinite peace and purposefulness that come with that.

And that's what I call "getting fit with faith." Think about the word *fit,* as in "It's a good fit." We all want to fit well into life—physically, socially, spiritually. When something fits, it becomes a natural part of the whole. It doesn't stick out awkwardly or draw attention to itself. It doesn't make you think about it. It just works.

Being physically fit is important, not just because it allows you to live longer and better, or because it makes others treat you better and improves how you feel about yourself, but because we inhabit physical bodies in the world and we don't want those bodies to limit our actions or our spiritual development. We want to have *unlimited* capacity for feeling God's love and for enacting that love. Your spirit needs to soar. And that means not letting it get dragged down by a body whose discomfort demands your constant attention. Part of having a fit spirit is having a fit body. It makes everything more joyful.

⌣ Activities ∿

Try any of these activities as a way of living purposefully.

- *When you walk today, pretend that your health depends directly on that walk. If you finish the walk, you will stay fit and healthy. If you don't, you will get sick or gain weight. Suddenly, that walk becomes quite urgent and purposeful! And truthfully, your health really is tied to that walk—it's just a long-term connection, and therefore harder to see.*
- *As you go through your day, ask yourself what the purpose was behind each of your actions or choices. Does each fit with your life's bigger purpose? What can you do to make more of your daily decisions on purpose?*
- *Plan out your day carefully, scheduling only things that fit your life's mission. When your day is filled with purposeful activity, you are less likely to get distracted by frivolous goings-on.*

⌣ Fit Facts ∾

Walk Away from Cardiovascular Disease

A half-hour daily walk reduces your risk of heart disease and stroke by 45 percent. By lowering your cholesterol and blood pressure, daily exercise keeps your blood vessels clean and flexible.

Time Yourself

The average American spends twenty minutes per day exercising and three hours watching TV. What about you? Do you see any imbalance here?

Priorities, Priorities

Ninety-one percent of American adults list good physical health as a top priority in life. Eighty-one percent list living with a high degree of integrity. Seventy-five percent list having a clear purpose for living. Seventy percent list having a close relationship with God. Nine percent list having the latest technology or gadgets. Six percent list achieving fame or public recognition.

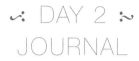

∙ DAY 2 ∙
JOURNAL

Walking on Purpose

Affirmation

"Every day I walk, I walk in devotion."

Today's Walk

How Far? _____

Strength Training? _____

How'd It Go? _____

Notes

_____

_____

_____

DAY 3

Speaking Truth to Power

Picture a little girl entering first grade. She goes out to the playground at recess and everyone is playing soccer. She's one of the youngest, has never played soccer, has no idea what to do, and no one's teaching her. And she's not as aggressive as some of the others. When the ball finally rolls her way, she misses it. She feels bad and some of her teammates give her a hard time. They stop passing her the ball.

The next day at recess, she gets picked last. Someone says, "Don't pick her; she's no good."

Pretty soon, the girl is avoiding soccer because it's an unpleasant experience for her. She never gets to practice and never gets better. If anyone asks her to play a sport, she says, "No, I'm no good at sports."

She—with a little help from her friends—has created a self-fulfilling prophecy. She believes she is no good at sports, hears others say it, and says so herself. Therefore, she may go her whole life avoiding physical exercise—all because of an idea that created its own reality.

How many of us have been that girl in some situation? If someone says you are bad at something, the pressure is on you to prove otherwise, and that's a pretty tough situation to be in. Most people excel at something when they are relaxed and expect to succeed. If you are expected to fail or expect this yourself, chances are you will.

You must expect to succeed. Whether your goal is getting fit or getting a promotion, whatever you expect to happen probably will—not always, but usually. And your expectations—your beliefs—come from what you and others say.

We like to think that we have a fixed set of beliefs, filed away in our head like books in a library. They sit there, unchanging, and we pull them out when needed. But in reality, our beliefs change all the time, even though we may not realize it. Thoughts are fleeting; they come and go like birds at a bird feeder. But once we speak something, that idea comes home to roost. The Bible says (Isaiah 55:10–11), "As the rain and the snow come down from heaven, and do not return to it without watering the earth and making it bud and flourish, so that it yields seed for the sower and bread for the eater, so is my word that goes out from my mouth: It will not return to me empty, but will accomplish what I desire and achieve the purpose for which I sent it."

Words create reality. They are "on the record" in a way that thoughts aren't. This is especially true if others are around to hear your words, but even if you're alone, what you say becomes what you believe. So be careful what you say!

If you wake up every morning, stare in the mirror, and grumble, "I'll always be overweight; it's in my genes. I'm not capable of exercising regularly," then I bet that comes true! On the other hand, if you say, "I've broken my patterns at last! I look better every day. I can't wait to exercise!" then you are going to be chomping at the bit to lace up those sneakers.

It's time for you to start speaking your reality into existence. It doesn't matter if you have trouble fully believing it at first. That part will come in time.

⌣ Having Faith ﹏

See if you recognize yourself in any of these un-faith-full thought patterns. Today, try to switch your inner dialogue so that your mind walks the walk along with your body.

Un-Faith-Full Thoughts:

- ﹃ I hate my body.
- ﹃ I'm sick of my spouse because . . .
- ﹃ I wish I had somebody else's life. Mine stinks.

⌣ Walking for Other Reasons ∿

*"He who guards his lips guards his life,
but he who speaks rashly will come to ruin."*
PROVERBS 13:3

Chances are that you've said something mean to someone, and then had to add, "Sorry, I didn't mean that." Then why did you say it? Sometimes two completely different people seem to be running our mouths and our brains! We think good thoughts, but somehow what comes out of our mouths doesn't always reflect them.

It's easy to get caught in the trap of saying critical things to family members or others we see all the time—including ourselves! This may be because we are tired and crabby, or it may be done sarcastically. But people can't see inside your head; they have only what you say to go on. Why not take the time to make sure what you say *is* what you mean, and that it's helpful? It doesn't have to be nice—sometimes things that are not nice need to be said—but it does need to be helpful, and true.

How can the things you say and do today further your goals? What connections can you draw between the integrity of your words (what you say to others and yourself) and how you treat your body? Do you always mean what you say? And if so, what have you promised your body?

⌣ Activities ∿

Try any of these activities today as a way of examining the way you use words—and the way words use you. If you find any of them helpful, keep doing them.

⚖ *Practice verbal leadership today. Pretend you are the president, or a minister, or some other leader, where everything you say is witnessed and acted on by many people. (Pretend this is true even when you're alone.) Does knowing that lots of people are looking to you for guidance change your words, thoughts, and actions? Did this raise your level of integrity? Why not speak with this level of integrity every day? (Remember, at least one person is always looking to you for guidance—you!)*

⚖ *If you don't want to be president, try being press secretary. Only instead of being press secretary for the White House, you are press secretary for God. Rather than respond with a knee-jerk reaction to somebody, take a moment to ask yourself, What would God's position on this be? Then stay "on message" in your response. You may discover a treasure trove of wisdom within yourself.*

⚖ *Pausing before speaking is a great practice in general. This is a lost art, and it seems strange to us if somebody stops and thinks for more than a few seconds before replying, but try it anyway. You may be amazed at how what you would have said changes, and deepens, when you give it time.*

⚖ *Look at yourself in a mirror and say three positive things about yourself, such as, "I'm energetic, capable, and self-confident." Look right into your eyes as you say them. Pretend you believe it. Pretty soon, you really will. And then it's true.*

⌣ Fit Facts ⌣

The Formula

To get a handle on your weight-loss goals, you need remember just one equation: Every ten calories consumed or burned on a daily basis equals one pound of weight per year. Drink one extra 150-calorie soda each day for a year and you'll gain fifteen pounds. Go for a vigorous two-hundred-calorie walk each day for that same year and you'll burn off twenty pounds. What small areas in your life can you change to tip this equation in your favor?

Be Careful What You Wish For

Percentage of college students who listed "financial success" as a primary goal: 74

Percentage who listed "having a meaningful life" as a primary goal: 43

Chromium Makes You Shine

Got the down-in-the-dumps munchies? Researchers have found that depressed people who take a daily chromium supplement cut their food cravings in half.

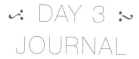

✌ DAY 3 ✌
JOURNAL

Speaking Truth to Power

Affirmation

"Walking makes me feel like a brand-new person.
I love to walk!"

Today's Walk

How Far? _____

Strength Training? _____

How'd It Go? _____

Notes

_____

_____

_____

A Witness for Fitness

Carol Best and Wayside Emmanuel Church
New Castle, Pennsylvania

My joyful walk with my Lord and Savior began in 1976, and my awesome health walk with Leslie began in 1996. Jesus saved and sealed my future; Leslie saved my to-days to witness for Him.

As an aging baby boomer, I had allowed myself to gain almost seventy pounds by 1996. Then my youngest daughter, Jolene, a kindergarten teacher at Spanish River Christian School, took me to a walking program taught by one of Leslie's instructors. Through much walking, guidance by Leslie's instructors, and knowing I could not be a testimony to any-one feeling sick, I have lost and kept off all of those nearly seventy pounds.

I am currently leading women at my church, Wayside Emmanuel, in an exciting journey of faith and fitness. What good are we unless we are fit for our Lord, families, and friends? Our testimony must be strong as our walk is strong with life. Leslie has a gift to share. As our Lord's gift of eternal life is up to us, so is our life's walk for fitness—it is a decision. Now, make your decision to walk the walk *every day of your life!*

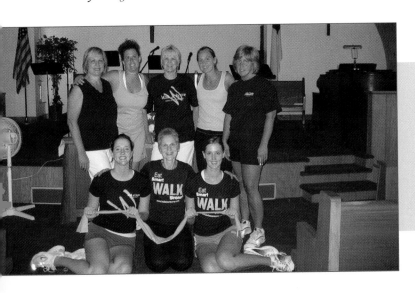

Getting a Hand from Above

For most of us, "alone" is not a great place to be. Eating alone certainly isn't much fun. Going to the movies alone always feels a little sad. Tennis alone? Not so great. Working alone can be great for concentration, but few people can do it every day. We crave fellowship. Living alone can be fun at certain stages of life, but even then we fill the emptiness with other voices on the radio and other faces on television. Being alone is not something many of us choose.

The tragedy is that we live in times of increasing isolation. Extended families live scattered across the country instead of clustered in a familiar town. Neighbors never introduce themselves. Workers telecommunicate. Those voices on the phone and those minds on the other end of E-mails must take the place of living and breathing human beings sharing a conversation in the same room. Sundays now are for mowing the lawn and watching football, not for worship and communion.

What does all this social isolation stem from? Just possibly, it comes from an even worse kind of isolation—estrangement from God. Many people today have lost their connection to God, and without that spiritual backing, the social tapestry starts to fray at the seams.

One casualty of this is our commitment to health. Why go to the trouble to eat right and treat our bodies well if we have no spiritual or social purpose? Sure, we know we should stay fit in order to make things easier on ourselves as we get older, but what's the point if there's no larger Point?

At the bottom of this slippery slope of questioning lies inertia. We stop taking care of ourselves, pushing our own needs aside. We may think about getting back on track, but it comes to seem like such an ordeal. As everyone knows, that first step is the hardest. If all the motivation has to come from us, it can seem nearly impossible.

Even if you manage that first step and begin a fitness routine, it's so easy to slip if you rely on willpower alone. An off day, a schedule conflict, and the first thing to get tossed is your exercise time. Willpower is only as strong as you are. When you're at your strongest, your willpower is, too, but you don't need it! You're on top of the world, feeling great, and exercise comes easily. It's when you're feeling weak that you need willpower to kick in and make you lace up those sneakers. But since willpower draws its strength from you, when you're weak, it is, too. If there ever comes a time when willpower will desert you, it will likely be at the worst time.

And that is when you sigh and say, "I can't do this alone!" And you're right. You can't. None of us can. Fortunately, you don't have to. There is a hand waiting to reach down, grasp yours, and lift you up to the place you want to be. It takes surprisingly little effort on your part once you make the life-changing decision to reach up and hold out your hand. That part takes some serious faith. A lot of people never get there. Until you admit your own powerlessness and open yourself to God's help, you aren't going to feel that help, so you aren't going to believe in it. But once you do, and you feel God take charge of your commitment, it becomes impossible to ignore.

This shift in focus seems subtle, but the effect is profound. Instead of waking up and asking yourself, What do I feel like doing today? you should ask, What does God want me to do today? Your relationship to the world and to your own motivation may change radically.

When you let God do the driving, a whole lot of things become easier. You don't need to worry about *why* you walk—you're walking for God. You don't need to worry about *if* you can do it—you can. He gives you the strength. He may not give you the strength to run a marathon right off the bat, because that isn't what you need. But He'll give you the strength to do what's right for you, and to keep getting better.

Whenever you feel like you just don't have the energy to stick to your goals—and everybody feels like this at some point—try asking God to step in and take over for a while. It doesn't hurt to really ask this—out loud. The walk on the DVD that comes with this book is another way to help bridge the gap. The inspirational music that accompanies it will set an uplifting mood that makes it easy to feel God's love and guidance. Remember, He is always there; it's up to *you* to find Him.

⌣ Having Faith ∾

See if you recognize yourself in any of these un-faith-full thought patterns. Today, try to switch your inner dialogue so that your mind walks the walk along with your body.

Un-Faith-Full Thoughts:

- ঌ I can't do this alone! I just don't have the strength.
- ঌ Nobody cares if I get overweight, sick, or depressed.
- ঌ I'm never going to be truly fit or thin, so I might as well just quit now.

Walking the Walk:

**"Thank you, Lord, for giving me the confidence and energy
to accomplish everything I set out to do."**

⌣ Walking for Other Reasons ∾

*"Rejoice in the Lord always. I will say it again: Rejoice!
Let your gentleness be evident to all. The Lord is near. Do not
be anxious about anything, but in everything, by prayer and
petition, with thanksgiving, present your requests to God.
And the peace of God, which transcends all understanding,
will guard your hearts and your minds in Christ Jesus.
Finally, brothers, whatever is true, whatever is noble, whatever
is right, whatever is pure, whatever is lovely, whatever is
admirable—if anything is excellent or praiseworthy—*

think about such things. Whatever you have learned or received or heard from me, or seen in me—put it into practice. And the God of peace will be with you."

PHILIPPIANS 4: 4–9

The Lord is near. How can we help ourselves to remember this through all our trials? If we do, and can feel that we are never truly alone, then we can begin to know true peace. Once we accept that everything is part of God's plan, then our anxiety about fixing things fades. Things will get fixed—or perhaps we'll realize that they were never actually broken in the first place.

But the challenge is to know this, to really know it, when it seems hardest to believe. The times we most need God are often the times when it is hardest to feel His presence. Think about the second part of the passage above. "Whatever is true, whatever is noble, whatever is right, whatever is pure, whatever is lovely, whatever is admirable—if anything is excellent or praiseworthy—think about such things." Simply thinking about that which is true and pure can help us escape a mental rut and reconnect with the source of divine goodness. It's always there, always ready to drop a rope ladder to help us climb our way out of the depths of a depression or grudge or anger.

Think about the things that get you into a funk. Instead of brooding on your own inadequacies or the unfairness of things and thinking that you will always be overweight/unfit/unhappy, what if you open your heart and mind to some of God's wonderful handiwork? Then you will feel yourself drawing near to Him. And the God of peace will be with you.

~ Activities ~

Try one of these activities as a way of reaching out and turning over your fitness commitment to God.

 ꝗ *Choose a talisman to get you in the mood for walking with God. This can be a favorite cross necklace, a special pin, or anything else lightweight that symbolizes your spiritual dedication. Save it for your walks or other exercises, or for other special times that require you to have strong faith. Whenever you put it on, you will immediately feel an intensifying of spirit. The talisman serves to elevate the occasion and put you in a mind-set that is receptive to God's presence.*

❧ *Use the DVD with this book to raise your walks to the level of worship. Our spirit is strengthened immeasurably when we carry worship with us outside a church pew.*

❧ *First thing when you wake up tomorrow morning, focus your mind and ask God to be with you throughout the day. Don't get up until you know you have truly reached out with your thoughts.*

⌁ Fit Facts ⌁

Big Belly, Big Trouble

Not all fat is created equal. Fat that you carry on your thighs and hips is closely connected with your natural weight and shape; it has little impact on your health. But belly fat isn't natural—it's a strong indicator of trouble. If your waist-to-hip ratio is higher than 0.8 (divide the measurement of your waist by the measurement of your hips to determine it), you have a high risk of heart attack. If you don't like your belly, it's time to step up to the next walking level.

The Satiety Index

Two foods that have the same number of calories won't necessarily fill you up equally. Depending on nutrient content and bulkiness, you can get a lot more satiety from certain foods, which means you'll snack less later on and consume fewer calories overall. The "satiety index" rates many common foods on their ability to keep you feeling full. The best: fruit such as oranges and apples (but not bananas), beef, fish, beans, eggs, oatmeal, whole-wheat bread and pasta, boiled potatoes, and popcorn. The worst: white bread, croissants, ice cream, cake, doughnuts, candy bars, and fried foods.

Walking's Better Than Dying

It's that simple: A two-mile walk five times a week reduces your chance of dying of a heart attack by 50 percent. Get walking.

Getting a Hand from Above

Affirmation

"I have everything I need for ultimate success. I'm tapped into the greatest source of energy in the universe, and today I will use just enough to get through the day with flying colors."

Today's Walk

How Far? _____

Strength Training? _____

How'd It Go? _____

Notes

_____

_____

_____

Being Thankful

Say it happens. You flick on the TV for the lottery drawing, pick up the ticket you bought yesterday, and watch in jaw-dropping amazement as first one, then two, then three, then four, five, and, yes, six of your numbers come up. You have just won $30 million! How do you feel?

Well, that's a no-brainer. *Spectacular* is how you feel. You scream, do a backflip over the couch, praise God, call your best friend, call your mother, gather the family, and take everyone you know out to dinner. Glory days are here. From now on, your worries are over and you will live in a state of constant bliss. Right?

Well, maybe not. Studies of lottery winners and others who have huge changes of fortune reveal that at first these people experience a surge of happiness. The bills are paid, the cars are upgraded, and it's prime rib for dinner every night. But then, after a surprisingly short time, most people return to their baseline level of happiness. This works both ways: Lose every penny in the stock market and you will be seriously bummed for a few months, but then chances are you will go back to feeling the same about life as you always have.

It isn't our external circumstances that set our level of happiness and contentment; it's our inner state. If you want to achieve lasting joy, don't bother buying lottery tickets; instead, work on your practice of giving thanks. You *did* win the lottery—the day you were born. We're all lottery winners. The prize: a life in God's loving embrace.

I can't think of a better way to be thankful for the gift of life than by engaging in some basic exercise. Exercise throws all the everyday worries out of our heads and reminds us of what's good: sweet air in our lungs, our faithful hearts pounding strongly in our chests, feet planting themselves one in front of the other. If you wonder why people who exercise regularly have such low rates of depression, wonder no more. Exercise helps us not to lose sight of the basics: Life is a blessing. In fact, when did we start calling exercise "working out"? Why does it have to be work? Let's take the *work* out of it and start "walking out" from now on!

After a nice vigorous three-mile walk, it's easy to feel thankful for God's gift of life. Your challenge is to take that postexercise glow and apply it to the rest of your life. You know how right it feels, how important, to go around the table at Thanksgiving and have each person say what he or she is thankful for. Why not treat every day as if it's Thanksgiving? (Just don't *eat* as if it's Thanksgiving every day!)

As you walk today, give thanks that you *can* walk. No matter where you are on your fitness or weight-loss goals, you have everything you need to achieve those goals. And that realization is pretty gratifying.

✌ Having Faith ∾

See if you recognize yourself in any of these un-faith-full thought patterns. Today, try to switch your inner dialogue so that your mind walks the walk along with your body.

Un-Faith-Full Thoughts:

- ↝ I have no luck at all. When will I ever get a decent break?
- ↝ I'm bored. Same old, same old. When do things get exciting?
- ↝ I guess God has given up on me.

Walking the Walk:

"Thank you, God, for the gift of a regular life. I promise not to waste it!"

⌇ Walking for Other Reasons ⌇

*". . . I have learned to be content whatever the circumstances.
I know what it is to be in need, and I know what it is to have
plenty. I have learned the secret of being content in any and every
situation, whether well fed or hungry, whether living in plenty or
in want. I can do everything through him who gives me strength."*
PHILIPPIANS 4:11–13

What is the secret to being content in every situation? We can find some clues in this scriptural quote: "I know what it is to be in need, and I know what it is to have plenty." Sure, we'd all rather have plenty, and we'd all rather be well fed than hungry, but knowing that we are going to experience some of each in life can help keep us from overreacting when the going gets tough. The ups and downs of fate are just that: ups and downs. An upswing will eventually be followed by some bad luck, and we may have a run of bad luck, when it feels like nothing will ever go right for us again—but it will.

An important part of learning to be grateful for every day is recognizing the separation between external events that happen to us and our eternal soul. Whether we lose a job or win the lottery, it doesn't affect our relationship with God. The poorest farmer in Africa is sometimes happier than the millionaire on Wall Street. This doesn't mean that the farmer wouldn't like an easier life, but it does mean that he derives pleasure and meaning from who he is and his relationship to the world and to God, not from what happens to him in the world.

This can be a hard lesson to remember. It practically needs to be relearned on a daily basis—every time something disappointing happens. What gets you down? Could it be that those disappointments are tests, part of the overall plan for your life? Do they really need to affect your contentment, or do you *let* them? As soon as you realize that you are giving them this power, you will be able to take it back from them.

༈ Activities ༇

Try one of these activities as a way to silence the whiny mind that can steal the joy from our days.

- ༄ *Make a list of everything you are thankful for. List* everything—*your family, your friends, your health, right down to tiny things like the bowl of ripe red strawberries you had for breakfast and self-adhesive stamps. The list itself is not important; you can even throw it out when you're done. The process is what matters; like any other skill, being grateful for the little things gets easier with practice.*
- ༄ *Switch lives. A great way to discover how good you've got it is to make drastic changes in your daily life for a day or even a few. You could swap chores with a friend, or could simply plan a day very different from your usual one. This often happens on vacation. As good as it is to escape the daily routine, we usually find that after a few days we start to appreciate our normal lives and are ready to return to them.*
- ༄ *Think back on the times in your life that you consider the happiest. What did they have in common, if anything? Was it circumstances that made you so happy, or was it some internal sense of mission or love or completeness? Identifying the internal state that generated your happiness may help you to stop pining for the "good old days" and to reclaim the state of mind that made them possible in the first place.*

༈ Fit Facts ༇

Alzheimer's and Diabetes

We have long known that diabetes raises your risk of cardiovascular disease by making it difficult for your muscle cells to receive the blood sugar they use for energy. Now researchers are learning that diabetes affects Alzheimer's disease for the same reason: With diabetes, brain cells lose their ability to process sugar, their only source of energy. This is just one more reason to avoid diabetes by exercising daily and eating a diet low in simple carbohydrates such as starches and sweets.

Really, Really Good Fat

Omega-3 is a special kind of fat found in fish, nuts, canola oil, flaxseed, and some whole grains. Just one gram per day of omega-3 reduces your risk of heart attack by 50 percent. It also reduces inflammation, protecting you against arthritis, cardiovascular disease, inflammatory bowel disease, lupus, and many other conditions.

It's Not the Money

Income and happiness have almost no relationship. Lottery winners and paraplegics rate themselves as being equally happy and optimistic. In a poll of workers, 80 percent of high-status workers and 75 percent of low-status workers called themselves satisfied with life. And while average income in America has surged since 1960, average happiness peaked in 1965 and has declined since. The only group that consistently scores higher in unhappiness is composed of individuals living in true poverty who can't meet their basic needs.

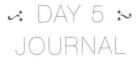
Being Thankful

Affirmation

"Today I appreciate the little things—
the roof above my head, the smiles of friends and family,
the great energy in my body as I walk."

Today's Walk

How Far? _____

Strength Training? _____

How'd It Go? _____

Notes

_____

_____

_____

DAY 6

Taking a Spiritual Inventory

The past five days, we've looked at ways to boost your commitment to fitness by calling on your faith. Today, let's shift gears and take a closer look at that faith. Faith is not a given, and one important goal of this book is to help you maintain it. Your faith can be neglected just as your health can. As with deteriorating physical health, dwindling faith often goes unnoticed for a long time before suddenly causing a crisis. If you don't exercise and you eat poorly, you start to develop cardiovascular disease. No one says the words *diabetes* or *heart attack* yet, but the damage to your arteries is slowly happening, and you don't even feel it except for maybe a little shortness of breath. Damage to your spiritual beliefs can be just as quiet. They slowly get eroded by a world that doesn't value spirit, but the damage is slow enough that you don't realize you're changing until a crisis occurs where you need to draw strength from your faith—and when you reach for it, it's gone.

That's why it's time to take a spiritual inventory—to see what you've got in stock and whether it's fresh or has reached its expiration date. Then you can decide if you need to do anything to fill up on faith.

The first question to ask yourself is, What do I really believe in? That's actually a tough question. We think we have a good handle on our beliefs until we need to verbalize them. Then the words don't come, because our core beliefs are locked away in a part of ourselves that is difficult to translate into words. But it's important to truly *know* our deepest beliefs, because they affect all our actions. Fortunately, this means that rather than try to state our beliefs in words, we can get a more accurate understanding of them by looking at our actions. Here are a few telling questions.

How do you treat your body? Do you consider your physical self sacred, or is it just a means to an end? Most people who abuse their bodies with bad food, cigarettes, or drugs have lost touch with their body's divinity. Even pushing your body too hard, overworking, or cutting back on sleep tells you a lot about your values—work or play first, health and stability last. Look back on how you've treated your body for the past week and, knowing that your body is the seat of the soul, consider what that means about your current relationship with your soul.

How do you treat others who have no power over you? Generally, we treat others pretty well when our fortunes are tied up with theirs—for example, bosses and coworkers, family and friends, doctors and teachers. It's in our self-interest. The more revealing question is, How do we treat all the others we encounter when there is no obvious reason for us to "play nice"? Clerks at gas stations and supermarkets, waiters, and customer-service reps are some examples. If we remember our shared fellowship and treat everyone in a way that would make Jesus proud, then we can be pretty sure our spiritual batteries are fully charged. But somebody who treats others as if they are disposable is not in touch with any sort of living faith. How have your interactions been during the past week? Could some of these have gone better if you had acted out of faith instead of insecurity?

Do you react to things off the cuff, or do you have firm principles that guide your reactions? If you don't act from a spiritual center, then every occurrence requires you to wing it, to take a stab at what you think might be right this time and make it up as you go along. Faith, on the other hand, provides a foundation of belief that makes most decisions quite simple. Think back on recent decisions you have made. Did you act with certainty or with doubt? If you have mixed feelings about what you are doing, then it probably isn't the right call. Generally, when you are truly on the Lord's path, moving in step with His wishes, you *know* it. You feel the deep clarity and peace inside that comes from there being no conflict between your spiritual core and your actions.

That doesn't mean you won't have doubts about your faith itself. You will, and you shouldn't feel guilty about them. An active, living faith is always marked by doubts. Any growing thing, whether a child or a tree, needs to be challenged in order to test itself and grow stronger. An unchallenged tree is a weak tree, apt to fall in the first real storm it faces. Similarly, a true, robust faith thrives on challenges. Having doubts is not a betrayal of your faith, or a betrayal of God. It's a recognition that your faith is strong enough to withstand anything the real world can throw at it; in fact, faith counts on such tests to pare away the weak parts so the living core can continue to develop and flourish. Question your faith whenever you want, but know that it is always there to help you to do the right thing.

Do you set aside times for worship? You can worship God in a million different ways. It doesn't have to be in a building with a steeple on top. It can even be inside your own head. But everybody needs to have some moments in their week that are purposely separated from the daily grind and devoted to higher thoughts. Every once in a long while, an intense spiritual revelation will hit like a lightning bolt; but most of the time, it takes a little effort to create a mental space calm enough to feel Spirit. Have you been getting these moments? If not, it may mean that faith has fallen off your to-do list.

This spiritual inventory could go on forever, but you get the idea. Ask yourself enough questions and look closely at your daily actions in order to get a sense of your true beliefs. What would you say those beliefs are? Do they need adjusting if you are to commit yourself to faith and fitness? If so, there's no better time than the present to take charge!

⌇ Having Faith ⌇

See if you recognize yourself in any of these un-faith-full thought patterns. Today, try to switch your inner dialogue so that your mind walks the walk along with your body.

Un-Faith-Full Thoughts:

- ⌇ I know I'm a spiritual person deep down, so it doesn't matter if people can't tell that from my actions.

- Faith is something you have or you don't. It's not something you need to work at.
- I have no time to think about spiritual matters. I'm way too busy.

Walking the Walk:

"God is a part of every step I take."

❧ Walking for Other Reasons ❧

"A simple man believes anything,
but a prudent man gives thought to his steps."
PROVERBS 14:15

Some people make the mistake of believing that their faith must be kept separate from the rest of their lives. They think that it shouldn't be sullied by being mixed up with the stuff of everyday life. But that is just where faith is most valuable—in providing a guiding light for daily decisions and challenges. Faith doesn't need to be kept on an altar; it's much more useful down on the street.

When you set up a wall between "real life" and the life of the spirit, you are more likely to let the spiritual life slip off your radar altogether. Then you have no guiding principle for your actions. What can you do to integrate your spiritual and mundane lives? For starters, give thought to your steps. Why are you walking the path you are?

Try to strike a balance between believing anything and believing nothing. You know there is some sensible place between these two extremes, where your faith informs your actions in the modern world but doesn't try to block out that modern world completely. That living, changing interaction between belief and experience is exactly what you want from a spirit-led life.

↵ Activities ∿

Try any of these activities as a way to better understand your own spiritual beliefs.

- ❦ *Write down your beliefs for right living. Keep this paper somewhere accessible, like in a day planner or on a nightstand. Review it once a day and, if you like, give yourself a grade for how well you've acted on your beliefs.*
- ❦ *Think about your parents' or grandparents' commitment to faith. How did it compare with yours? Can you see reasons why they developed as they did? How did the decisions they made influence your own beliefs?*
- ❦ *Set your watch or cell phone to go off every hour during the day. When it does, think of the most recent decision or action you made, small or large. Does it fit with what you think of as your beliefs, or is there a disconnect between what you say you believe in and how you act?*

↵ Fit Facts ∿

Take Art to Heart

Several studies have shown that regularly experiencing art, whether it's music, literature, or paintings, reduces your blood pressure and makes you happier and more creative.

Nursing for *Your* Health

Here's some more good news for new moms. Most of us have heard how breast-feeding gives babies a terrific head start in life, from boosting their immune systems to protecting them against diarrhea and malnutrition, but it turns out nursing is just as good for the mother. It removes stress hormones from your system, lowering blood pressure and increasing relaxation. It reduces the risk of diabetes by 15 percent for each year of breast-feeding, because it lowers blood sugar. Think of nursing as intense exercise: You burn five hundred calories a day doing it, only instead of those calories being used to power muscle, they are powering your baby. Nursing may even cut your risk of breast cancer in half.

Keeps Away More Than Vampires

Along with vampires and coworkers, a few of the things you can keep away with a regular dose of garlic are clogged arteries, high cholesterol, high blood pressure, and some cancers.

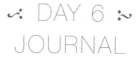

Taking a Spiritual Inventory

Affirmation

"I am a whole, seamless person.

Everything I do today will be a perfect reflection of my beliefs."

Today's Walk

How Far? _____

Strength Training? _____

How'd It Go? _____

Notes

_____

_____

_____

A Witness for Fitness

Cathy Manning
Smyrna, Georgia

In November 2001, I weighed in at my doctor's office at 281 pounds. I was in shock. As I left the office, I knew that I had to do something about my weight. Each new morning, I pledged to start a diet; every night, I ate enormous amounts of foods. By the beginning of 2002, I tipped the scales at three hundred pounds. I could walk down steps only if I held on with both hands and watched my feet land on each step. I'd long stopped fitting into airplane seats. Office chairs were miserable, as the arms cut into my thighs. My grocery bills were growing by leaps and bounds.

My sister arrived for Christmas fifty pounds lighter. I decided if she could do it, I could also. I ordered Weight Watchers At Home kit. I got up every morning and started counting points. When the points were gone, the kitchen was closed.

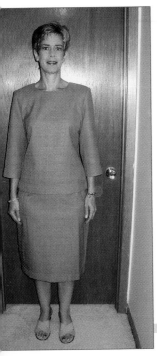

From the very beginning of my journey, I knew that exercise was important to my success. One day, on a Weight Watchers site board, I read about Leslie Sansone and her Walk Away the Pounds program. I headed straight for the store and bought the videos. I recall begging Leslie to stop about seven minutes into that first mile. Thank goodness she couldn't hear me! With her persistent enthusiasm, she kept right on walking, kicking, and sidestepping. Not being a quitter, I determined that I'd keep up with her one day.

Before long, I moved on to Leslie's two-mile video, then her three-mile one. When I discovered that Leslie had an abs series, I bought that. What fun a new workout was! What a pleasure to be able to keep up with Leslie and her walkers! I had pictures of me taken in my workout clothes as I lost the pounds and toned my muscles. Each morning as I walked, I saw where I'd come from, and I envisioned where I was going.

Eighteen months later, I met my goal. I'm half the size of my highest weight. Gone is my closet of multisize wardrobes. I have only clothes that fit, with the exception of one of my "fat dresses" as a reminder of where I came from. I continue to exercise at least five days per week, and I watch what I eat.

There were times along my journey when I thought that I couldn't go on another day. But God had other plans for my life. When I'd think I couldn't go on, I'd find a verse from Scripture like Psalm 46:1: "God is our Refuge and Strength (mighty and impenetrable to temptation), a very present and well-proved help in trouble." What a blessing to have found an eating plan and an exercise plan that worked for me. And three years later, I still get excited when I spot a new Walk Away the Pounds workout DVD in the store . . . and I probably always will!

Self-Love

We are beautifully and wonderfully made! Yet too many people out there think of their bodies as a problem rather than a joy. It's easy to see why this is so. Every day we are bombarded by advertisements telling us that our looks don't measure up in some way, and that we need new products to compensate. Or we see gorgeous models and actresses and know that we *don't* measure up—at least not to the airbrushed images we are shown. Or we have modern lifestyles that demand little from our bodies, feed them too much, and thus allow them to deteriorate to a state we never would have chosen and don't like the look of. Often this state includes health problems that limit us or cause us discomfort. The upshot is that the body becomes a source of anxiety and embarrassment instead of comfort. Soon, we hate our bodies and everything associated with them, and that can quickly morph into self-hatred for the person that goes with the body.

This, of course, is not what God intended. He created you as a spiritual being in a physical world and expects you to have love for all His creations, yourself included. You are part of His plan. You don't need to worry about whether you are fulfilling God's plan for you. It's *His* plan, after all, not yours! All you need to do is be true to yourself.

I remember when I was a little girl of five or six, getting ready for my First Communion. A nun told my mother that things had changed and girls didn't all wear white anymore. Well, my mother seized on that. She went out and bought me the cutest bright yellow dress you'd ever see. And there I was, posing for pictures in church on Sunday—one yellow dress amid a sea of perhaps a hundred white dresses! My mother was mortified and wanted to get ahold of that nun. I could also have felt like I stuck out, a black sheep (or a yellow one), and been humiliated, but I wasn't. I felt beautiful. It didn't even occur to me to worry what anyone else thought. I was so excited to be taking Communion, so proud, and that was all that mattered.

God made you to be human. To serve Him, you simply need to live a proper human life. Be good to God. Be good to your planet and your community. And be good to yourself. That includes loving your body as it is right now. You must accept your body and make friends with it. If you are at odds with it, you are never going to be able to "get on the same page" with it and work toward your wellness goals.

You may be thinking, But why should I love my body? It causes me nothing but grief! But that's not how love works, is it? Your kids sometimes cause you grief, but you still love them, right? True love is unconditional. And that's how God loves you. God has invested much in you. Jesus invested *everything* in you. If they feel such love for you, how can you not feel it, too? They are counting on you. They would never give up on you, and you must not, either.

We all tend to develop an image of ourselves and then turn it into a self-fulfilling prophecy. If you tell yourself, I'm shy, then you'll act that way, too. But if you tell yourself, I have fun meeting new people, then chances are that you will. If you see yourself as a lazy person, then you have the perfect excuse to not do much! But if you see yourself as a high-energy achiever, then chances are very good that when given the opportunity to achieve, you'll take it! In this way, we all "think" our own destiny into being.

It never feels good to be fighting yourself, or to be fighting your destiny. What feels good is being part of the team, marching in step. In this case, the team is your mind, your body, your spirit, and God. If there is some tension between any parts of this team, call a team meeting now and get it out in the open. You can't trade away any of these players, so learn to love them. Then you will find out how they excel when entrusted with your faith and given the chance to perform. Before long, you will be a winner every day!

◡ Having Faith ◡

See if you recognize yourself in any of these un-faith-full thought patterns. Today, try to switch your inner dialogue so that your mind walks the walk along with your body.

Un-Faith-Full Thoughts:

- ❧ I'm a nobody. I'll never accomplish anything important, so what's the point in taking care of myself?
- ❧ I hate my weaknesses and my habits. There's something wrong with me.
- ❧ My spirit is pure. If only I didn't have this dumb body to lug around, everything would be perfect.

Walking the Walk:

**"I feel the divine spark in my body and soul
and do everything I can to further God's plan."**

◡ Walking for Other Reasons ◡

"Woe to him who quarrels with his Maker, to him who is but a potsherd among the potsherds on the ground. Does the clay say to the potter, 'What are you making?' Does your work say, 'He has no hands'? Woe to him who says to his father, 'What have you begotten?' or to his mother, 'What have you brought to birth?' "
ISAIAH 45:9–10

In recent times, we, as a society, have gotten into the dubious habit of constantly questioning our lives. Should I change jobs? Should I change congregations? Should I move? Is my marriage good enough? Is my nose good enough? Spend enough time analyzing anything and you're sure to stop enjoying it. Sometimes it's better to spend less time questioning and more time accepting and moving forward.

As I said earlier, it's normal to have doubts about your faith from time to time, but that's no excuse to reject God's gift of life and body. God created you to be a human being, and questioning that would be as silly as a clay bowl questioning why it is a bowl. You have a purpose to fulfill, just like that bowl. Take the tools God has given you, love them, and use them to serve Him well.

⌣ Activities ∿

Try any of these activities as a way to renew your self-acceptance.

- ✽ *Pretend your body is your child. If your child was getting out of shape due to poor eating habits and lack of exercise, and getting down on herself because of the emotional and social problems this was causing, how would you treat her? Would you say, "You're right, you really are a jerk"? Of course not! You would tell her that she was special, that you loved her no matter what, and that with a little work she could be exactly like she wanted to be. And you'd know it was all true! Counsel yourself like a wise parent would. Love yourself like a wise parent would.*

- ✽ *Make a list of all the things about yourself that drive you crazy. "Plans to eat one cookie but eats ten." "Gets the french fries instead of the side salad." "Thinks about walking first thing in the morning, then hits the snooze button and sleeps an extra hour instead." Pretend you are on trial and that you have presented the list to the judge. What would the punishment be? Self-torture? No, exercise! Now, get out there and take your "punishment."*

- ✽ *Find a picture of yourself that you really like. It should be one that makes you smile inside when you see it. It doesn't matter how old the photo is, even if it's from when you were a kid. Post it on your fridge and look at it every day. You still are that person! Love yourself like you do that person. Act like that person.*

∿ Fit Facts ∿

Weighing Muscle Versus Fat

As you continue your walking routine, you may find that after a few months the scale doesn't drop each week as quickly as it used to. Does this mean you're slacking off somehow? Not at all! Muscle weighs more than fat, and the more you walk and do strength training, the more muscle you build. So just because the scale isn't budging doesn't mean you aren't looking better every day. Don't let the scale lord over you; instead, check your measurements, especially waist and hips, or dress size. Better still, just look in the mirror. If you feel like you're looking better, you most definitely are!

Go High-Pro for Weight Loss

More and more scientific studies show that low-carb, high-protein diets like South Beach work better for weight loss than low-fat diets. In one recent study, volunteers on a high-protein diet were able to eat 441 fewer calories per day than volunteers on a low-protein, high-carb diet.

Dark Chocolate—Rich But Not Sinful

Dark chocolate is packed with antioxidants known as flavonoids, which lower your cholesterol and blood pressure, keeping your blood vessels clear and flexible and reducing the risk of heart attack and stroke. Milk chocolate has more sugar and fat in it than dark chocolate, so it has no positive impact on health. Stick to the dark stuff—look for labels that say the product contains at least 60 percent cocoa.

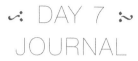

DAY 7
JOURNAL

Self-Love

Affirmation

"I am a creation of God's love, excellence, and beauty."

Today's Walk

How Far? _____

Strength Training? _____

How'd It Go? _____

Notes

_____

_____

_____

DAY 8

Finding Compassion

When you think back to the most meaningful moments in your life, they aren't always the easiest moments. Meaning often comes in situations where your character develops by being tested in some way, or where you suddenly understand a new life lesson for the first time. More often, our truly meaningful moments involve compassion—either we reached out to someone else in their time of need or they reached out to us. Either way, a bond was formed and a trouble eased because of compassion.

We can all agree that compassion is an important Christian virtue, but the goal of this book is getting fit with faith. You may be thinking, Come on, Leslie, compassion and fitness are totally separate. One has nothing to do with the other. Yet I believe they have *everything* to do with each other. If you have been struggling to achieve your fitness goals, finding compassion may be the thing that boosts you over the top.

Many people out there know the loneliness that comes with feeling really bad about themselves. You get out of shape; your energy is low. Far from compassion, about the only feelings you sense coming your way from other people are disappointment, disapproval, and distancing. That all makes it harder to turn the corner and begin climbing your way back into shape, walking the walk and losing those extra pounds. Compassion can be the key to turning that corner. If you feel as though no one cares what happens to you, it's harder to care yourself. But if you feel buoyed by a sea of supporters, if you know that others out there are pulling for you and cheering your every success, you aren't going to disappoint them, and you aren't going to disappoint yourself.

Now, here's the tricky part. How do you find that compassion? If you simply keep searching for it, you may not find it anywhere. You'll feel like compassion has been blotted from the earth! No, the secret to finding compassion is giving it!

Maybe you have been treated badly by others in your life and you closed down in response. It's understandable; if all you receive from others is pain, then why keep receiving? But once you close down to meaningful sharing with others, you can't receive love, either. And you can't *give* love or compassion or anything else. Maybe you worry about being taken advantage of, about sending out too much compassion and not getting enough back, until eventually your compassion runs dry. But compassion never runs dry. It is a limitless well. The more you send out, the more it wells up within you.

Think about the people you know who seem to show endless compassion to others. Maybe it's a family member, maybe a minister, or maybe just a very good friend. You marvel at how their generosity never stops; they always seem to have more and more love in them. And maybe you have been reserving your own love, parceling it out in dribs and drabs as if it were an oil supply you didn't want to run out. If that's the case, the time has come to open those pipelines wide and let it flow. It will never cease, but only grow stronger. You've got a gusher connecting straight to God, the original source of compassion.

And don't forget about the rebound effect. The more compassion you have for others and put out into the world, the more will flow back to you. With your channels of love and communication wide open to others, you will suddenly see that the compassion you couldn't find before was there all along, waiting for a way to reach you. Some people are utterly convinced that no one out there is waiting to offer them compassion; they are the ones most surprised and gratified to find it flowing strongly to them from sources they never could have imagined. The key to the equation is flow: The more powerfully you put it out there, the more powerfully you'll receive it.

Back to fitness. On this eighth day of your commitment to getting back on God's plan for you by getting your body up to speed, think about ways you can start creating compassion. Don't worry about *who* is going to give you the compassion you need; just think about who might need yours and be sure to send it. Who could benefit from a reminder of how much you love them? Find a total stranger and make their day in some small way. That act of opening yourself to the world will assure that nothing is blocking compassion from reaching you. And when you feel that compassion come your way and fill you with a warm glow, use that energy to break through to a new fitness milestone so that you'll have even more energy and joy to return to the world tomorrow.

✌ Having Faith ∿

See if you recognize yourself in any of these un-faith-full thought patterns. Today, try to switch your inner dialogue so that your mind walks the walk along with your body.

Un-Faith-Full Thoughts:
- ∽ I expect nothing from others, and they shouldn't expect anything from me.
- ∽ I don't need anyone's help or love. I can do it all myself.
- ∽ It's us versus them.

Walking the Walk:
"We are all a part of God's plan and all deserving of love."

✌ Walking for Other Reasons ∿

"Finally, all of you, live in harmony with one another; be sympathetic, love as brothers, be compassionate and humble. Do not repay evil with evil or insult with insult, but with blessing, because to this you were called so that you may inherit a blessing."
1 PETER 3:8–9

What is compassion? It's not simply being kind to others; you can hold a door for somebody without necessarily feeling compassion for them. Compassion is a deeper feeling than kindness; it requires being able to put yourself in another's place and understand the common ground you share. It's about making a connection with another human being—and that connection is God. That's why compassion has always been a basic part of being a Christian. God links us all; finding compassion is simply grasping this and acting on it. Because it's not enough to simply feel it; you must act, too. By acting on your compassion, you further God's plan.

To be compassionate is to never be alone. You are part of a compassionate universe. As the Bible says, Christ lives in you. You never feel this blessing more than when you allow love to flow.

Who out there needs your love and sympathy and isn't getting it? Who could you give an emotional boost to today? What friendships have you let slip, and what's to stop you from making that call today and bringing that relationship back to a state of harmony and blessing?

∿ Activities ∿

Try any of these activities as a way to recharge your compassion batteries.

- *Do something unnecessarily nice for a total stranger. When the person in front of you at the coffee shop is fumbling for correct change, hand it to her. Then use that good feeling to propel you through your next walking session with an extra lift in your step.*
- *Make a surprise visit, or at least a phone call, to a friend or elderly relative. When the person asks why you are calling, say that you were just thinking about her and wanted her to know how much she means to you.*
- *Ask your friends and family to add your health goals to their prayers. As you work toward fitness, think of them out there offering you their compassion.*

༈ Fit Facts ༈

Hypnotic Healing

Hypnosis—putting someone in a state of mind where he or she is perfectly focused on a single thought and is unaware of the outside world—is proving surprisingly effective in terms of health. It helps wounds to heal significantly faster, is almost always successful in treating skin conditions, reduces severity of headaches, and allows most people to feel much less pain from chronic conditions—including cancer, where those who use self-hypnosis even live longer. It also has proved very helpful in achieving life goals.

Dr. Dog

Forget the physician; if you want to stay healthy, put your trust in Fido! People who take up dog walking lose an average of fourteen pounds in a year. People who go on typical food diets lose about six. But dog benefits go beyond that. Pet a dog and feel your stress-hormone levels drop by a quarter. Ahhhh . . . I mean "woof!"

Don't Diss Dairy

Dairy products have a bad rap right now, due to the news that saturated fat is a main culprit in incidences of heart disease and stroke. On top of that, many people believe they are lactose-intolerant and can't eat dairy products. But dairy products can be an excellent part of a healthy diet. People who eat a lot of *low-fat* dairy products tend to lose more weight than people who consume the same amount of calories but eat fewer dairy products, because the high protein content of dairy products encourages feelings of satiety. Dairy products also provide one of the best sources of calcium, a key mineral for preventing osteoporosis (decrease in bone mass). In addition to protein and calcium, dairy products provide many other vitamins. And even people who are lactose-intolerant can eat yogurt. Look for low-fat or no-fat dairy products, such as skim milk, to avoid artery-damaging saturated fat.

Finding Compassion

Affirmation

"Today I will feel God's love shining through me
and say a blessing for everyone I meet."

Today's Walk

How Far? _____

Strength Training? _____

How'd It Go? _____

Notes

_____

_____

_____

Building Strength

Say you're having a moment of weakness. The world is weighing heavily upon you and you can barely stand the pressure. "God, give me strength," you pray. And He will—though not always in the way you expect. One of the ways God keeps our spirits strong is by giving us the means to build our own strength. Strength training is the best way to do that. It involves exercises quite different from aerobic ones such as walking or running. Strength-training exercises are usually short, quick moves repeated many times, such as lifting weights, doing crunches, and pulling against rubber resistance bands. These moves increase your muscle power: When muscles are challenged, they become bigger and stronger, so they'll be up to the challenge. That process provides a whole goody bag of benefits, some going well beyond the obvious physical ones. Here's a highlight list.

1. Great looks. If you see somebody with awesome tone, you know they are doing some sort of strength training. Words like *tone* and *definition* are really just code words for *muscle*. Muscle, unlike fat, retains its form even when not being used. It ripples, while fat *sloshes*. And nothing builds muscle like strength training. Walking helps you burn calories, prevents cardiovascular disease, boosts your mood, and makes your muscles more efficient, but, unlike strength training, it doesn't make them bigger. Don't underestimate the importance to your spirit of having a strong, solid body! It's not a matter of showing off or being vain; it's just a question of having the confidence to engage life boldly, knowing your body won't let you down or embarrass you. And that's all for the good!

2. **Preventing osteoporosis.** Osteoporosis happens to most women as they age. Does this mean it's inevitable? Not at all! The reason it happens to most women is because most women don't exercise, especially when they are older. Bones are not the permanent building blocks we think they are; our bodies must constantly reinforce them with new calcium, which is the "mortar" they are made from. That's necessary because bones steadily lose calcium through natural processes. It's the pull of working muscles on bone that signals your body to reinforce that bone and make it stronger—and nothing creates that pull like strength training. If your body doesn't feel that pull, it assumes those bones aren't so important, and then they leach calcium and become porous and brittle, more likely to break under pressure.

3. **Fewer accidents.** It's good to have healthy bones that are less likely to break in a fall, but it's even better not to fall in the first place! Strong muscles allow you to do all sorts of activities with confidence, and they are there for stability when you miss a step or slip in the snow. This may not be a big issue when you're forty, but you'll appreciate it when you're sixty, and love it when you're eighty!

When people tell me they have reservations about strength training, it usually comes down to one of two things. Either they don't like gyms or weight machines or they are already walking with me for half an hour every day and can't squeeze any more exercise time into their day. Fortunately, I have a solution to both problems! My style of strength training is done right at home, with no expensive equipment, and it doesn't take a single extra minute of your time! The secret? You do it while you walk, using simple hand weights or stretch bands. Even doing the motions without weights or bands helps. Your walking sessions become more fun and more productive.

"All right, Leslie, I'm convinced. I'll try some strength training. But how do I get started?" you may say. Glad you asked! Simply pull the DVD from the inside back cover of this book and follow my arm motions along with the walking. Just like that, you're doing strength training!

ꞈ Having Faith ꞈ

See if you recognize yourself in any of these un-faith-full thought patterns. Today, try to switch your inner dialogue so that your mind walks the walk along with your body.

Un-Faith-Full Thoughts:
- As long as my faith is strong, I don't care what happens to my body.
- The body is an evil source of temptation. I wish I could separate myself from it.
- Paying attention to my body is a shallow thing to do.

Walking the Walk:
"I will do what it takes to stay strong into my ripe old age, because I have many important things to do while on Earth."

ꞈ Walking for Other Reasons ꞈ

"Do you not know that your body is a temple of the Holy Spirit, who is in you, whom you have received from God? You are not your own; you were bought at a price. Therefore honor God with your body."
I Corinthians 6:19–20

You want to live in a strong, solid house, right? But why? So your house can be the envy of all the other people who live on the block? So it can be tougher than the other houses? Of course not! You want a solid house because that building is the foundation for most of the activities that go into a healthy, fulfilling life. Family and friends gather in the house. Rest and relaxation happen in the house. Creativity and inspiration and love fill the house. Your house is your sanctuary, your place of entertainment and socializing, your tool for everything you want to do in life. That's why it's so important to have a strong house that is pleasing to you. If you can't spend time with your family because you are devoting all your waking hours to a leaking basement, a sagging roof, and peeling paint, if you can't create art or run your business at home because the walls and furnishings are demoralizing and the refrigerator acts up all the time, or if you can't experience love or faith because you are preoccupied by drafty windows and soaring utility bills, then your house is preventing you from living life to the fullest.

Now think about your body. Your body is the house for your spirit; it's your temple for receiving God. You need to keep it sound and well maintained, just like your house, so that you can receive His love without the distractions of a dilapidated body. If you ever feel selfish devoting time to working out, remember that you are not your own property, and the Landlord is going to be thrilled by the changes you are making!

Activities

Try any of these activities as a way to work strength training into your routine.

- *Today, think of your body as a house that God is coming to visit. What can you do to spruce up the place and prepare for the visit?*
- *Don't want to use any equipment for strength training? Try Pilates! This revolutionary technique uses special postures to make certain parts of the body work against one another or against gravity, creating natural resistance. It's easy and effective! (My Pilates DVD is a great place to start.)*
- *Do strength training while you work. While at your desk, tie a stretch band to a chair leg and your ankle and stretch it out and back for ten minutes. Then switch to the other leg.*

⌣ Fit Facts ∿

Young Bones

Women in their seventies who do regular strength training have bones that are just as strong as they were when these women were in their thirties. Women who don't do strength training lose from 1 to 2 percent of their bone mass each year, starting when they are in their mid-thirties.

Keeping the Burn Going

Vigorous strength training burns about six calories per minute—only about half as much as vigorous aerobic exercise. But strength training raises your body's metabolic rate—the rate at which you burn calories—for an amazing fifteen hours after a one-hour workout!

Reducing Menopause Symptoms

Reaching menopause doesn't mean it's too late to begin exercising! In a recent study in Spain, women ages fifty-five to seventy-two who completed a yearlong program of aerobic, strength-training, and relaxation exercises had just half the rate of severe menopausal symptoms that nonexercisers did. They also had much improved mental states and quality of life.

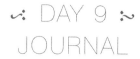

Building Strength

Affirmation

"Each day I get stronger,
and each day I get a little closer to God."

Today's Walk

How Far? _____

Strength Training? _____

How'd It Go? _____

Notes

_____

_____

_____

A Witness for Fitness

Carolyn Duckworth

Beacon Evangelical Free Church, Galloway Township, New Jersey

Leslie's years of hard work and dedication to walk aerobics inspired me to start the walk aerobics class at my church, Beacon Evangelical Free Church, in Galloway Township, New Jersey. Our class used to consist of nine ladies, and now it's up to about thirty. We meet Monday through Thursday, 9:30 to 10:30 AM, and do a two- to four-mile walk, with Leslie as the instructor, thanks to our collection of her DVDs and the big movie screen, projector, and sound system we use for our church services. Our church sanctuary is a multipurpose room, so it's great for walk aerobics. After the walk aerobics, we have about fifteen minutes of prayer, praises, and Scripture devotion. This has been a great opportunity for outreach missions and fellowship. We are taking care of God's temple (our bodies) in God's house. Moms bring their babies, too, and get a great workout. What a great testimony! We have so much fun! We especially love the inspirational three-mile cross-training walk.

My personal testimony is that my husband is in the Pomona Air National Guard and is in Iraq now, serving our country. I have a goal to lose weight before he gets home. Working out with other women motivates me to want to be there. We are in the best house (God's) and we are building relationships and taking care of our bodies for free. *Amen. Come and visit anytime; our doors are open.*

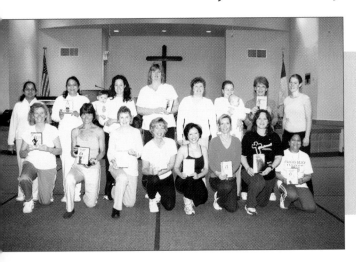

Sacred Food

Eating is a wholesome act. It goes to the core of what it means to be alive. So it only makes sense that we thank God by saying grace before a meal, for food is a constant reminder that we are blessed and that life is interconnected.

But how should a good Christian eat? Certainly not the way so many of us do. You know the routine: After church, we get together for a table laden with sweets, mac and cheese, soft drinks, potato salad—the carbohydrates of the world. Christians take a great deal of pleasure in making food and in breaking bread together, but somewhere along the way, the types of food we once ate changed drastically, with serious implications for our health—and our faith.

It's simply a lot easier to forget that food is sacred when you pick it up through a drive-up window than when you grow it yourself. When you raise your own food, it's hard not to see the life burgeoning in the plants and animals, and to see God as the source of all that life. Saying grace comes naturally.

But in the twenty-first century, fewer and fewer of us are still connected to these natural life cycles. We still go through the motions of saying grace, still try to be thankful whenever we think of it, but it's easy to forget the bigger picture when all of our food is prepackaged and served up by one corporation or another, and rarely resembles the plant or animal it came from.

If this were just a matter of being thankful, it would still be important, but the implications go much deeper: because the same processes that result in convenient packaged food also result in disease. Losing touch with the sacred nature of food leads us to lose touch with health, and most of the time we aren't even aware of it.

The simple fact of the matter is that the closer foods are to their natural state—to the way God made them—the better they are for us. The human body developed before the era of machines that could strip the outer hull off of grains, pulverize them, and reconstitute them as chips and cookies. It developed before catsup was considered a vegetable. It developed before trans-fats, corn syrup, and saccharine, and before animals were injected with antibiotics and growth hormones.

Your astonishing digestive system can take a piece of raw broccoli and break it down into tiny bits of fuel in just a few hours. That's pretty power-ful! In fact, your body is happiest when it gets foods in fairly natural states: fresh vegetables, whole grains, and naturally cooked meats. Like a kid gnawing on an apple, your digestive system takes a while to break down such foods into the tiny molecules of sugar that can be burned for energy—mean-ing your blood sugar stays nice and level.

When, instead, you give your body white flour, white sugar, or other processed foods, where machines have done most of the work of break-ing the food down for you, your body is able to absorb it much too fast—and thus blood sugar rises. Eat that way long enough and you will develop diabetes.

Processed foods also tend to contain much more unhealthy saturated fat than whole foods. And saturated fat is a leading cause of heart disease and stroke.

It's one thing to know which foods we shouldn't eat, but where do we look for a model of how we should eat? Look no further than Jesus, the ulti-mate role model for so many behaviors. Jesus lived in the Mediterranean re-gion, of course, and the popular Mediterranean diet, touted by so many health organizations for its ability to reduce the risk of heart disease, cancer, and many other illnesses, is pretty much how Jesus and his contemporaries ate every day.

The Mediterranean region of Jesus' day was a farming area. Grains, fruits, and vegetables made up the bulk of most people's diets. That's still true in Greece, Italy, and the other Mediterranean countries, and it's the foundation of the Mediterranean diet. The diet sounds complicated, but its rules are actually really simple:

1. Eat mostly fruits, veggies, and whole grains.
2. Eat fish, poultry, eggs, beans, and nuts as your main protein sources.
3. Use olive oil as your main fat source.
4. Eat sweets, starches, red meat, and whole-fat dairy products sparingly.

That's it! Follow those four rules, along with the guideline to try to eat foods in their natural states as often as possible, and you'll be home free. The benefits include not just weight loss but also a significantly reduced risk of diabetes, heart attack, stroke, and cancer. I covered nutrition thoroughly in my previous book, *Leslie Sansone's Eat Smart, Walk Strong,* but here are some very brief explanations of the benefits of a balanced diet:

1. Fruits, veggies, and whole grains: These provide vitamins and fiber. Vitamins are the tools the body uses to do all the tasks it needs to stay healthy, and fiber isn't digested by the body, so it fills you up without adding calories. The result: You eat fewer calories overall, lose weight, and stay healthy.
2. Fish, poultry, eggs, beans, and nuts: These provide protein, which your body needs to build and maintain strong muscles, bones, skin, organs, and the nervous and immune systems. If you get your protein from red meat instead, it comes with lots of saturated fat, which causes cardiovascular disease.
3. Olive oil: This oil provides healthy fat. Contrary to popular belief, fat does not make you fat. A modest amount of fat is essential to good health. It makes you feel full faster, so you eat less at meals, and healthy fat also lowers your cholesterol levels. The saturated fat found in red meat and dairy products is the bad stuff; it raises your cholesterol levels and clogs your arteries.

4. **Sweets and starches:** These are both simple carbohydrates, which get turned into blood sugar right away. This contributes to diabetes and hardening of the arteries. And when your blood-sugar level drops, you get hungry, so spiking your blood sugar with soft drinks or french fries sets you up for the munchies in an hour, when your blood-sugar level starts to come down. That's why simple carbohydrates are the leading cause of obesity—people who eat them can't stop.

5. **Red meat and whole-fat dairy products:** As mentioned above, these clog your arteries and lead to heart attacks and strokes.

Sacred eating—eating the foods that God put on the good Earth for us—keeps you on the straight and narrow path to lifelong health without having to think about it. On this tenth day of your monthlong commitment to walking His walk, take a few moments to renew your eating vows, too.

↭ Having Faith ↝

See if you recognize yourself in any of these un-faith-full thought patterns. Today, try to switch your inner dialogue so that your mind walks the walk along with your body.

Un-Faith-Full Thoughts:

↫ I don't have time to eat a healthy meal. I just need to shove something down because I have important things to do.

↫ I hate food because it makes me fat.

↫ Who cares if I eat this pint of ice cream instead of dinner? No one will even know.

Walking the Walk:
**"I know God is always with me when I eat,
helping me get the energy I need to serve His kingdom."**

⌁ Walking for Other Reasons ⌁

"So whether you eat or drink or whatever you do,
do it all for the glory of God."
1 CORINTHIANS 10:31

Imagine you stop at a convenience store, buy a jumbo bag of potato chips, say grace in your car, then chow down on the entire bag. You'd feel pretty silly, wouldn't you? Thanking God for the potato chips would feel false, because you'd know you were about to do something harmful to yourself—something God didn't want you to do. You may have plenty of reasons why you need to pound a bag of potato chips at that moment, but doing it for God is not one of them.

What if you really did do all your eating and drinking for the glory of God? What would your diet be like? It would be full of foods that would keep you healthy, because God wants us all to be healthy so we can do His work. It would probably be full of foods obtained from farmers who were doing their part to raise healthy crops and livestock and keep the Earth holy. And it would probably be in the company of other people as often as possible, so you could share His love when you shared His food.

Now, the question is, Why *don't* you always eat or drink for the glory of God? Could you? Should you? Would you benefit from doing so? What do you have to lose by trying?

⌁ Activities ⌁

Try any of these activities as a way to begin your path of healthy eating.

༄ *Say grace before all your meals. Whether you have everyone at the table partici-*
pate or you just do it silently doesn't matter; do whatever's comfortable. Any way

you do it, thanking God for your food will put you into a new relationship with it; you'll see it for what it really is. Is it sacred food, or low-grade entertainment?

❧ *Start a vegetable garden. It doesn't need to be big; just growing some tomatoes and basil is a good way to start. What a perfect way to remind yourself how much love goes into growing food! If you have kids, let them help; they'll be making deep connections that will serve them well their whole lives.*

❧ *Volunteer at a soup kitchen. It's easy to take food for granted when we have plenty. Volunteer at your church's soup kitchen and you'll serve some people who most definitely do not take food for granted. You'll realize that the gift of food is precious.*

∿ Fit Facts ∿

You Have a Friend in Fiber

Fiber sounds too good to be true—a nutrient that fills you up but has *zero* calories. But it is true. Fiber can't be digested by the body, so it fills up your stomach while it's in there but then passes on through. It also absorbs water, which causes it to bulk up, making you feel fuller on fewer calories. Studies show that women who eat high-fiber diets (at least twenty-two grams per day) have very little chance of being overweight. And that's why high-fiber diets are associated with a reduced risk of diabetes, cardiovascular disease, and some cancers. The best foods for fiber are fruits, vegetables, legumes, and whole grains.

Fish for Your Heart

Eating fish just once or twice per week can cut your risk of heart attack *and* colorectal cancer by a third! The reason? Fish is high in heart-healthy omega-3 fatty acids, and when you're eating fish, you're *not* eating artery-clogging, colorectal cancer–inducing red meat.

A Better Breakfast

If you are one of those people who nibbles a bagel in the morning and calls it breakfast, you might not be doing yourself any weight-loss favors. Researchers measured the total daily calories consumed by women who ate a 340-calorie breakfast of a bagel, cream cheese, and yogurt versus those consumed by women who ate a 340-calorie breakfast of eggs, toast, and jelly. The women who ate the bagel breakfast ended up consuming an average of 274 more calories during the day than the women who had the egg breakfast. Why? The combination of protein and healthy fat in eggs makes you feel full longer than if you ate a bagel, which is high in refined carbohydrates.

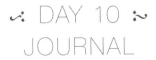

JOURNAL

Sacred Food

Affirmation

"Today I will put nothing but God's
natural foods in my glorious body."

Today's Walk

How Far? _____

Strength Training? _____

How'd It Go? _____

Notes

_____

_____

_____

Sacred Drink

Baptisms are among the loveliest of church ceremonies. A new babe, as pure as pure can be, gets a sprinkling of water and begins life in a state of grace. But there are so many interesting liquids out there, why does it always have to be water? Why not baptize with a mocha latte, or maybe a can of Red Bull?

What, you don't like that idea? There's something about the water that fits? I admit it: I agree! Nothing but water can symbolize the clean state of a new soul. No drink but water is associated with life itself, which is why water is the only sacred drink there is.

And well it should be. Without water, no life is possible. Human beings are basically water balloons with legs and arms. Our bodies are two-thirds water, and some organs, such as the brain and kidneys, are more than 80 percent water! Virtually every function of our bodies depends on water. Food gets broken down with saliva; nutrients, energy, and hormones get distributed through the blood; antibodies circulate through the lymphatic system; heat gets dispersed through sweat; and so on. Go a couple of days without water and this all breaks down.

Even a mild case of dehydration has unpleasant consequences. Unfortunately, many of us go through most days mildly dehydrated and don't even know it. Some of the first signs of dehydration are fatigue, headaches, and irritability—sound like anyone you know? A national campaign to get everyone to drink eight glasses of water a day could do wonders for the health and morale of all Americans, and eliminate the consumption of a lot of unnecessary caffeine and pain-killers.

Eight glasses a day is a good general guideline for how much water you should drink. (Remember, we're talking six-ounce glasses, and most of today's glasses are much larger than this, so don't think that you need to chug eight tumblers a day!) Do this and you'll have more energy (because water is responsible for ferrying fuel to your muscles and brain), fewer health problems (for example, water makes up 80 percent of your cartilage, which cushions all your joints and prevents arthritis), and better skin.

Anyone who has kids has come up against the primary objection to drinking water. "Aw, Mom, water is boring!" You may even think this yourself. If so, you have lost perspective. Is air boring? Is love boring? Don't take it for granted just because it needs to be a constant in your life.

You can substitute milk, juices, or soft drinks for water and meet your fluid needs, but along with that liquid, you'll be getting hundreds of calories a day, which can add up to twenty, forty, or even sixty pounds a year! Switching to water for most of your drink needs is one of the easiest and most effective ways to diet imaginable. Diet drinks are okay, and you can jazz up your water with a squeeze of lemon or with bubbles, but why not try pure water? The more regularly you drink it, the better it tastes—and the more cloying soft drinks taste. After awhile, only water will supply that sacred purity you thirst for. Best of all, water is abundant—like God's love.

◡: Having Faith :◡

See if you recognize yourself in any of these un-faith-full thought patterns. Today, try to switch your inner dialogue so that your mind walks the walk along with your body.

Un-Faith-Full Thoughts:

- ↷ It doesn't much matter what I put in my body. Coffee, soda, iced tea—it's all the same.
- ↷ I know I need to stay hydrated, but I don't see anything so special about water, and I don't see how it could connect to faith.
- ↷ As long as I work out regularly, I can eat and drink anything I want and still stay fit.

Walking the Walk:
"With every glass of water I drink, I am bathing my soul in God's goodness."

⌣ Walking for Other Reasons ⌣

*"Jesus answered her, 'If you knew the gift of God
and who it is that asks you for a drink, you would have asked
him and he would have given you living water.'*

*" 'Sir,' the woman said, 'you have nothing to draw with and the
well is deep. Where can you get this living water? Are you greater
than our father Jacob, who gave us the well and drank from
it himself, as did also his sons and his flocks and herds?'*

*"Jesus answered, 'Everyone who drinks this water will be
thirsty again, but whoever drinks the water I give him will
never thirst. Indeed, the water I give him will become in him
a spring of water welling up to eternal life.' "*
JOHN 4: 10—14

In this well-known story, when Jesus tells the woman at the well that he would have given her living water, he is referring to the Spirit of God and eternal salvation. He could not have chosen a better metaphor for this than water. Think back to some point in your life when you were really, really thirsty. Maybe you were walking on a blistering day. Or maybe you were on a long drive and had no water in the car. Think back to that time and remember how, after awhile, all you could think about was water. Once you get thirsty enough, fantasies about Coke or coffee fly out the window and you want just one thing: clear, cold water. Now think about when you got it. You tipped that cold glass or bottle to your mouth and let the good water splash in. That rush of well-being that comes with this is not like the feeling we get from savoring the flavor of a food or drink; it's more like the satisfaction of restoring a part of ourselves that was missing—which is the truth. And that's why Jesus' metaphor was so perfect. Accepting the gift of eternal life for the first time is to realize that a part of ourselves was lost and has been found; it is to realize that we've been thirsty all our lives and have drunk from the deep, cool spring at last.

Ritual is a way of using mundane acts to remind ourselves of profound truths. Every time you fill up with a glass of life-giving water, use it as an opportunity to remind yourself of the living water that washes your soul.

⌣ Activities ∿

Try any of these activities as a way to begin purifying your body and soul with water.

- *Drink a glass of water before you get thirsty. That means one in the morning when you wake up and more throughout the day whenever you think of it. Drinking lots of water (cool but not ice-cold, which can hamper digestion) with your meals will help you stay hydrated and allow you to fill up on less food.*
- *Drink a glass of water before and after exercising for maximum performance. Your energy is less likely to flag halfway through a walk, and you'll find you can walk farther and burn more calories.*
- *To remind yourself of water's sacred role in life, make it feel sacred. Maybe drink only natural springwater. Or maybe you have a beautiful glass that has special meaning to you and can become your exclusive chalice for the life-giving elixir.*

⌣ Fit Facts ∿

Creep, Creep

The average adult gains one pound a year, starting around age eighteen. That doesn't sound like much, but it means twenty extra pounds when you're forty, and forty extra pounds when you're sixty. The way to beat the creeping weight gain? Cut just ten calories from your daily diet. Drinks are often the easiest place to start.

Watch Liquid Calories

You'd think that a calorie is a calorie is a calorie, but not according to the body. Some calories keep you full (because they come in fat or protein, which take a long time to digest) and some don't. Sugary drinks are absorbed very quickly into the bloodstream, leaving you as hungry as ever. For every two calories you consume in drinks, you cut back on solid food by only one calorie. That can leave you consuming hundreds more calories per day than you wish.

Beware of Sneaky Water

There are now hundreds of waters on the market that have flavors or are fortified with extra nutrients. But often they come with a nasty little present, as well: lots of unnecessary calories. Make sure your water has zero calories—and get those nutrients through healthy foods instead, like fruits and veggies.

Sacred Drink

Affirmation

"Today I commit to drinking water with
my meals and before and after my exercise."

Today's Walk

How Far? _____

Strength Training? _____

How'd It Go? _____

Notes

_____

_____

_____

Pay Attention

Say you commute to work every day along the same route. Generally, you're racing along at sixty miles per hour, gnawing on a bagel and wishing the slowpoke in front of you would get vaporized by aliens so that you could speed up. But today, you break down two miles from work. You've gotta walk the rest of the way. For the first few minutes, you stew about how late you'll be and the meeting you'll miss. You can't *believe* how long it takes to cover ground at a walking pace! And if you don't get to work soon, you won't outperform everyone else, and then you won't get ahead and get raises, and then you won't be able to retire early so that you can do things like . . . take a walk whenever you want.

After awhile, you surrender to the fact that you can't make yourself go any faster, and you trudge on. Then you notice the flowers by the side of the road. They're quite beautiful, like tall blue sunbursts. Have they always been there? Strange that you never noticed them before. It's a sunny morning and you feel the pleasing warmth on your cheeks as you walk through a residential neighborhood. You pass a lovely old house and wave to the retired couple sitting on the porch. You smile as you see them enjoying their morning together. By the time you make it to the office, you are filled with an unexpected peacefulness from the things you have witnessed and the accomplishment of your two-mile walk.

What you have just done is pay attention to the micromoments that make up the here and now. You'd never have noticed them if not forced by circumstance. You've passed through those moments at warp speed a hundred times, so obsessed with catching up to the future that you were incapable of registering their existence, much less enjoying them.

Learning to pay attention to what exists in the moment is one of the best things we can do to achieve faith and fitness. Does God exist more strongly in that future moment you are striving toward than He does in the present one? Of course not. Then what is so great about that future moment? God is all around you right now, emanating from every object and person, including *you*. Paying attention to that fact doesn't mean doing anything about it; it just means being aware of it. And being fully present in the moment doesn't mean not planning for the future, but it does mean not putting off your own peace and contentment until some future time when everything will be perfect.

Think how much stress and energy is wasted worrying about the future or the past. A classic example is when you lie awake at night, obsessing over the coming day. Through the wee hours of the morn, you toss and turn, worrying about this or that "unsolvable" problem. Then it occurs to you that you aren't getting your needed sleep and you're going to be tired and useless the next morning. Now your fear of not sleeping is keeping you awake! Why not simply lie there and pay attention? There are times when you would *kill* for two hours to do nothing but lie peacefully in the quiet dark.

There are no boring moments, only failures of perception. Something extraordinary is *always* happening. A caterpillar is turning into a butterfly. Your child is catching a ball for the first time. You just rescued a spider and set it free outside. You just baked your first loaf of bread. If the ultimate goal of life is to receive and give God's love, to experience heaven on Earth, can't you achieve that right now?

How can paying attention affect your fitness success? By teaching you that walking is not a means to an end. If the sole reason you walk is to lose weight, you are going to come to resent that half hour of your day pretty quickly. But walking is an end in itself! It's fun and it feels right, because your body was made to walk. If you enjoy walking on its own terms, you will keep doing it every day, and many other achievements will simply fall into place—including a beautiful body, mind, and spirit.

༄ Having Faith ༄

See if you recognize yourself in any of these un-faith-full thought patterns. Today, try to switch your inner dialogue so that your mind walks the walk along with your body.

Un-Faith-Full Thoughts:

- ༃ I wish I'd started walking earlier and was twenty pounds lighter by now.
- ༃ I have no time for myself or my family right now; I need to work 24/7 to get that raise!
- ༃ This is boring. I wish I were somewhere else instead.

Walking the Walk:

"I am exactly where I need to be right now. Everything is all right."

༄ Walking for Other Reasons ༄

"My lover spoke and said to me,
'Arise, my darling,
my beautiful one, and come with me.

See! The winter is past;
the rains are over and gone.

Flowers appear on the earth;
the season of singing has come,
the cooing of doves
is heard in our land.

The fig tree forms its early fruit;
the blossoming vines spread their fragrance.
Arise, come, my darling;
my beautiful one, come with me.' "

SONG OF SONGS 2:10—13

When we're falling in love, we get especially good at noticing the small miracles of life: the cooing of doves, blossoming flowers, the beauty of a rainstorm washing over the land. Everything seems to be ripe with purpose. Everything we do, whether picking fruit or walking, is for our loved one.

If we are in love with God, we can hold this feeling in our hearts all the time. What can you do to capture that excitement of new love and carry it with you? What beauty do you witness? What joy do you take in everyday tasks such as cooking, working, and walking? What can you do to spread this joy to others?

⌁ Activities ⌁

Try any of these activities as a way to keep your mind from wandering into the past or future.

- ❧ *Have a spouse, friend, or colleague buzz you at random moments throughout the day. When they do, take full stock of your surroundings and what you're doing and thinking. What was going on around you or inside your own head that you weren't even aware of? The more you do this, the more aware you'll become.*
- ❧ *Keep a daily list of beautiful things. In my first book,* Walk Away the Pounds, *I suggested noting moments or things of beauty in your day, however small, and writing them down, and the idea has proved to be very popular. Doing this helps train the mind to see the beauty that is always there.*
- ❧ *Walk, don't drive. Trade in the car for some sneakers when doing some errand. Yes, it's going to take you longer. Accept that, plan accordingly so that you aren't anxious, and enjoy the time. What do you notice on foot that you would have missed in the car?*

༈ Fit Facts ༉

Eating with Your Eyes

When it comes to hunger and satiety, the eyes are every bit as powerful as the stomach. Consider this clever study: Researchers had volunteers eat bowls of soup, half of which were in secretly self-refilling bowls. People eating soup from the refilling bowls ate 73 percent more soup, but they estimated that they had eaten the same amount as the people with the regular bowls, and judged their fullness the same, as well. Other studies show similar results. People eat 45 percent more popcorn from bigger boxes and drink a third more from wider glasses. The upshot: We tend to eat most of whatever we're served. The solution: Use small glasses, bowls, and plates and you'll eat less without even realizing it.

Nature's Tylenol

People who engage in regular brisk walks or other exercise feel 25 percent less joint pain than sedentary people.

Watch Out for Transfats

Transfats—oils made to have improved shelf life by bubbling hot hydrogen gas through them—are the deadliest type of fat. They usually go by names like hydrogenated vegetable oil and are found in all kinds of crackers, chips, and baked goods with long shelf life. Cutting transfats out of your diet will cut your risk of cardiovascular disease in half. Cutting them out of the American diet could save tens of thousands of people from fatal heart attacks. Now that transfats are required to be listed on nutrition labels, you may think you can steer clear of them, but don't forget about the biggest source of transfats: fast-food french fries and fried chicken. A serving of McDonald's french fries has a whopping twenty-three grams of transfats, while their chicken has eleven grams. KFC isn't far behind. A better choice is a grilled chicken sandwich with a salad on the side.

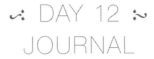

⌣ DAY 12 ⌣
JOURNAL

Pay Attention

Affirmation

"Today is today, and I embrace it with all my will."

Today's Walk

How Far? _____

Strength Training? _____

How'd It Go? _____

Notes

_____

_____

_____

A Witness for Fitness

Cheryl Janusek
West Mifflin, Pennsylvania

As a Catholic Church secretary for over twenty years now, my walk in faith is a daily one. My faith was what enabled me to begin my health journey so many years ago. I had developed asthma and needed to quit my habit of two and a half packs of cigarettes a day. On my lunch break one day in 1987, I walked over to the church and prayed to Him to take away my desire to smoke. Miraculously, I stopped smoking that very day! I knew if He led me to quit smoking, He would again guide me in weight loss.

Nineteen eighty-seven was also the year I turned the dreaded four-oh. My best friend had asked me to be her matron of honor, and the idea of walking down the aisle at 240 pounds in a size twenty-four-and-a-half dress was more than I could take. I decided to try Weight Watchers, and prayed to Him to get me through it. I knew I could not do it alone. By 1988, I had lost ninety pounds and reached my goal. Then the hard

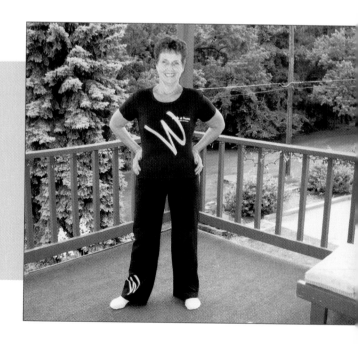

part began! Losing the weight was fairly easy; maintaining my new weight was far more difficult.

I had not learned how big a part exercise and activity play in weight management. I did the least I could. I just never found any form of exercise that I enjoyed enough to be consistent about. The only exercise I half-liked was walking, but when it rained or snowed or was too hot outside, well, no exercise for this gal! Then, *one day in 1997, I watched Leslie Sansone demonstrate her walk aerobics. After a few minutes of trying it, I thought, Gee, this is fun. I have been walking with Leslie ever since. Her program enables me to exercise whenever I choose, no matter the time of day or the weather outside. Not only has Leslie's program enabled me to maintain my weight but, at fifty-nine, I have more energy, stamina, strength, flexibility, and muscle tone than ever before! I am healthier and feel better than I ever have in my life.*

I have been blessed with a wonderful family and friends, all of whom have always shown their support on this life's journey of mine. And now with three grandchildren to romp with, I am easily able to keep up with them. I've gone from a person who was content to stay in the background and let life go by to a person who loves life and all its challenges!

I feel privileged to be able to help others on a daily basis with their fitness journeys, spreading the word of good health and physical fitness. I lead a walk class in our parish twice weekly, and what a diverse group it is, from an eleven-year-old to those in their eighties! We literally throw up our hands and thank God for our good health. We not only get our spiritual fitness here at St. Joseph Parish but our physical fitness, as well. As Leslie tells us, "It's all connected!"

Healing Dis-Ease

Your natural state is one of ease, comfort, and joy. This shouldn't be a momentary feeling you get while taking a bath or eating a really good piece of chocolate; you should feel this way most of the time. As spiritual beings in physical form, we should be able to draw on God's love whenever we need it, to dwell in it every day. If we can't access that state, then something is wrong. Something is blocking our spiritual reception. And the consequences to our health are astonishing.

Before the development of modern medicine, Western doctors believed that good health was a matter of balance. If you kept the body's systems in balance, you stayed well. Eastern medicine has held similar beliefs for thousands of years and still does: Keep the body's energies flowing and you keep sickness at bay. When negative energy gets blocked in the body, it manifests as illness.

We don't need to accept this idea hook, line, and sinker to acknowledge that inner unease is linked to physical disease and discomfort. Stress shows up as tension in your back or temples. (More on the physical effects of that on Day 25: "Outfoxing Stress.") Spiritual malaise shows up in the way your shoulders droop, the way you drag yourself through the day.

Just as a plant needs sunlight, your body and soul need the light of God to shine in them. If that light is blocked, you droop as surely as a plant kept in the dark. If you are frequently ill, or rarely feel joy in your days, ask yourself the reasons. Is the culprit your physical environment, your spiritual environment, or a combination of the two? The two are related in many ways. If you have an ear infection, there's a clear physical culprit (though it certainly affects your spirit, too). But if you feel like you have chronic discomfort, if you simply don't feel good in your body, then your "leaves" may not be getting enough spiritual light. Time to dust them off.

As you walk today, try to let all your mental discomfort go. Usually about fifteen minutes into a good walk, we forget other concerns and lose ourselves in the pleasure of moving. You already know that regular cardiovascular exercise helps prevent physical disease; today, remind yourself that it also restores mental ease. And that kind of inner comfort is your birthright!

∿ Having Faith ∿

See if you recognize yourself in any of these un-faith-full thought patterns. Today, try to switch your inner dialogue so that your mind walks the walk along with your body.

Un-Faith-Full Thoughts:

- ∿ Why am I always sick?
- ∿ I feel like I just got run over, but I've gotta keep doing the daily grind.
- ∿ Life is work. It wasn't meant to be all fun and games.

Walking the Walk:
"Life is good. I really look forward to each day."

∿ Walking for Other Reasons ∿

*". . . Whoever listens to me will live in safety
and be at ease, without fear of harm."*
PROVERBS 1:33

It's a fact that churchgoers live much longer than nonchurchgoers. Why do you think that is? Are they being rewarded for their attendance? Or does making that extra effort to connect with the divine source bring an incredible sense of comfort and fulfillment that translates into better health? Whatever the reason, we know that making the effort pays incredible dividends.

What other ways can you introduce inner peace and joy into your life and the lives of those you love? One way to think about this is to look at what blocks your joy. There are all the usual stressors—which we'll consider in Day 25—but there are also the deeper issues of spirit. Knowing that you are true to God and true to yourself gives you the confidence you need to laugh off annoyances as just that. They are annoyances, but they quickly fade away.

For many of us, our bodies are a primary source of unhappiness. We don't like the way they look or the way they feel. We worry about getting older and losing our health. We think, That's not me. I'm trapped in someone else's body! And there's no escaping this body that makes us uncomfortable, so there's no peace.

But remember the proverb on the previous page: "Whoever listens to me will live in safety and be at ease, without fear of harm." Remember that, and be at ease! You are taken care of. There is nothing to worry about, so why not take care of your body? Knowing that you can live without fear, and that you can do everything you need to take care of your body, allows you to operate from that place of peace and security that makes it so easy to make the right decisions.

∽ Activities ∾

Try any of these activities as a way to reclaim your sense of ease.

⚘ *Try a visualization exercise. When you have a quiet moment, close your eyes and picture yourself as a tree. Visualize your leaves unfurling all around you, and imagine a golden light falling upon them. As the light hits you, feel the comfort and joy filling you. Breathe deeply and relax, knowing that this is your natural state. Remember these feelings so that you can access them whenever you need to during the day.*

8 *Give yourself a "spa" day. Devote twenty-four hours to your physical well-being. Eat incredibly healthy foods. Get exercise. Get an aromatherapy foot treatment. Avoid cigarettes, caffeine, and alcohol. Do anything else you can think of to create a sense of supreme healthiness.*

8 *If you have any chronic health conditions or annoyances, trace back to when they started. Was there some change in your life that coincided with the change in your health? What can you do to change any current habits that you suspect are affecting your well-being?*

⌣ Fit Facts ∾

A Prayer a Day Keeps the Doctor Away

Churchgoers have greater life expectancy than nonchurchgoers, and the more often you go, the longer you can expect to live!

Attendance	Life Expectancy
More than once per week	83
Once per week	82
Less than once per week	80
Never	75

Sssshhhh

On average, every six decibels of increased background noise will raise your blood pressure a point. That's why living in a very noisy city neighborhood can *triple* your risk of heart attack! Choose quiet spaces for working and sleeping.

Kicking the Habit

Churchgoers are more likely than other people to successfully break free from bad physical or mental habits.

Problem	Percent by which churchgoers are more likely to break free of mental conditions or physical habits compared to nonchurchgoers
Depression	131%
Smoking	78%
Being Sedentary	54%
Alcoholism	39%

Healing Dis-Ease

Affirmation

"My natural state is abundant joy, health, and well-being.
When I wake up in the morning, this is the first thing I feel."

Today's Walk

How Far? _____

Strength Training? _____

How'd It Go? _____

Notes

_____

_____

_____

DAY 14

Looking Good Is Not a Crime

What's the single thing that can improve people's looks the most? High-heeled shoes? A six-month diet? Actually, for my money, I'd say nothing beats a smile. A smile can take a gloomy face and make it look younger, prettier, more confident, and, of course, much, much happier.

Consider the people you think generally look good. Chances are they aren't superskinny. They probably don't look like models. Most likely, they are somewhat fit, fairly well put together, and they are almost always wearing a smile. Are you one of those people?

True good looks are the outer reflection of a healthy spirit, mental state, and physical body. Inner health and happiness can't help but show through— in a person's body, in how she presents herself to the world, and in how she takes care of herself by eating right, exercising, and by acting in a way that says she respects herself and her place in the world.

There is no crime in making the effort to look good. Too many of us feel that somehow we don't deserve to look good, that it's selfish to spend time on ourselves that could be devoted to others. We somehow think that if we deny ourselves anything nice, then we are being more virtuous. But when you make yourself feel good through just a touch of pampering, when you treat yourself to a new piece of clothing and feel excited to wear it, when you take the time to do your daily walk, you improve your spirits tremendously, and you will be far more likely to seize the day with terrific energy and do everything you can to further God's plan for you. Others will thank you, and you'll thank yourself.

On this day, as you near the halfway point of your monthlong commitment to fitness, go the extra mile to put your best face forward to the world.

See if this improves the way others treat you, the way you feel about yourself, and the success this positive outlook brings to your day.

✧ Having Faith ✧

See if you recognize yourself in any of these un-faith-full thought patterns. Today, try to switch your inner dialogue so that your mind walks the walk along with your body.

Un-Faith-Full Thoughts:
- ✧ I'm going to stay in my sweats all day today. Who am I trying to impress?
- ✧ Either you're attractive or you're not. New makeup, clothing, and hairstyles can't make a difference.
- ✧ I can't force a smile. I just don't feel it inside.

Walking the Walk:
"As God's servant, I try to represent Him as I think He'd want me to. He smiles through me."

✧ Walking for Other Reasons ✧

"Your beauty should not come from outward adornment, such as braided hair and the wearing of gold jewelry and fine clothes. Instead, it should be that of your inner self, the unfading beauty of a gentle and quiet spirit, which is of great worth in God's sight."
1 Peter 3:3–4

The wise speakers of the Bible caution us against focusing on outer adornment rather than an inner virtue, and it's good advice. No amount of ornamentation can compete with "the unfading beauty of a gentle and quiet spirit." And vanity is certainly a sin. But notice that the preceding biblical passage doesn't say that you should avoid adornment entirely; it just says it shouldn't take the place of what is infinitely more important in God's sight.

Does the beauty of your spirit shine through? If not, what can you do to let it? Given the chance, inner beauty will express itself in someone's face, in how she carries herself, and in the entire style she presents to the world. That's what Peter is urging. Let your outer package be a perfect match for your inner self. If you have a spirit that is strong, fit, and graceful, then your body and style will come to be the same if you let them.

When our inner and outer selves *don't* match, we feel tension. In some way, we are living an untruth. We may become frustrated when we feel that we have a vibrant soul that is trapped in a body that just won't get it together. When that happens, there must be some external factor preventing you from leading the lifestyle that your body naturally wants. If you feel a lack of harmony between what you feel in your soul and what you see in the mirror, see if you can identify the factors that might be responsible. What changes can you make so that your unfading beauty is clear for all to see?

⤳ Activities ⤶

Try any of these activities as a way to give yourself the best self-image possible.

- *Plant a smile on your face first thing in the morning and leave it there all day. Not a big Bozo the Clown smile, just a pleasant, subtle, closed-lip smile will do. After awhile, you'll feel more positive about your day, and others will react to you by smiling back. It's contagious!*
- *Treat yourself to a piece of clothing you've been wanting, or maybe a makeover. If this makes you feel good about yourself, use that energy to walk farther than usual or to do something else positive for yourself and the world.*
- *When you dress in the morning, pretend you are going to be giving a presentation on the power of faith. As God's representative, what will you wear? How will you act?*

༈ Fit Facts ༈

Low-Fat Diets Don't Work

The low-fat diets that became popular in the early 1990s don't work. The latest evidence comes from the huge Women's Health Initiative Dietary Modification Trial, which tracked the eating habits of 49,000 women. Twenty thousand women ate a low-fat diet, reducing their fat intake from 38 percent to 20 percent and getting diet counseling from those conducting the trial. The other 29,000 women ate their normal diets. After eight years, the two groups had no difference in weight or rate of cardiovascular disease, breast cancer, or colorectal cancer. All these risks are reduced, however, by switching your intake of saturated fat to unsaturated fat, such as that found in fish, vegetable oils, avocados, and nuts.

Lactic Acid—Your Muscles' Best Friend

Forget everything you thought you knew about lactic acid. For years, we've been told that lactic acid is a waste product generated by muscles as they burn glucose, and that it's the source of the burn you feel after hard exercise. Now scientists have discovered that lactic acid is fuel—made by our muscles on purpose! Mitochondria, the little power plants in each of our muscle cells, would rather burn lactic acid than anything else. When you push yourself to your exercise limits, that causes your muscles to make more mitochondria—meaning you'll burn lactic acid more efficiently the next time out and will go farther before running out of steam. What really does cause that postworkout burn? Scientists don't yet know.

A Yogurt a Day Keeps the Doctor Away

An exploding field of medical research is the study of probiotics. Found in food, these microorganisms act like security forces in your gut, keeping the bad microorganisms out. And it is now thought that those bad microorganisms are linked to a lot more than the occasional upset stomach; they may play a role in everything from cancer to colitis and Crohn's disease. A steady supply of probiotics may help prevent these diseases or reduce their symptoms if they are already present. A Swedish study found that people taking probiotics were less than half as likely to take a sick day as people who weren't. Best places to find probiotics? Any yogurt or kefir (a type of yogurt drink) that says "contains live cultures" on the package. Probiotics are also available as dietary supplements.

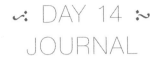
Looking Good Is Not a Crime

Affirmation

"With each step I take, I'm on my way to being healthier, happier, and more attractive than I've ever been!"

Today's Walk

How Far? _____

Strength Training? _____

How'd It Go? _____

Notes

_____

_____

_____

Tiptoeing Past Temptation

Your warm bed instead of church on a Sunday morning, the tub of ice cream instead of the navel orange, the Food Network instead of the walking DVD—temptation lurks everywhere! It's a slippery rascal, always whispering in your ear, telling you to do something you know you shouldn't. Like an annoying relative, it often shows up unexpectedly—especially at holiday time!

How do you defeat temptation? Let me be the first to tell you that you can't. Sorry, it won't work. You can throw out all the junk food in the house, buy yourself lots of exercise equipment, join three churches and pray to live free from temptation, but temptation is still going to find a way to slip into your house and play its mind games on you. Temptation can't be killed. Even if you've been good for years, sooner or later you are going to slip.

But don't despair just yet. In this case, you don't need to defeat temptation to achieve victory. You just need to keep it down to a dull roar. A little temptation won't hurt you; temptation wins only when you allow your small slipups to weaken your spirit. A strong spirit can take whatever blows temptation delivers and stay on its life path without wavering, but a wounded spirit can get derailed by temptation and may sometimes take years to get back on track.

How do you stay strong in the face of temptation? By learning to live with it. This is one more case where laughter really is the best medicine. When you laugh at temptation, it loses all its power. Laugh at yourself. When you treat yourself with amused and loving fondness, knowing that you are going to have a few setbacks mixed with your victories and that this is all part of your journey, then you don't get demoralized, and temptation can't achieve too much power over you.

I call this chapter "Tiptoeing Past Temptation" because it's best not to tackle temptation head-on. Don't take the job at the candy factory! Don't get an alarm clock with a snooze button! Don't wake temptation any more than necessary; sneak past it instead. You know it's going to get you now and then, so don't give it extra chances.

What happens when temptation does get you? Laugh, shake it off, and get right back on your path. You may have walked two miles for three weeks straight; then you catch a cold and don't walk two days in a row. Does that mean you're a disaster and you should abandon your goals? Of course not. It means you're human! You are *allowed* to slip up. You are *expected* to. As long as you don't make it a habit, you'll be fine.

✍ Having Faith ∿

See if you recognize yourself in any of these un-faith-full thought patterns. Today, try to switch your inner dialogue so that your mind walks the walk along with your body.

Un-Faith-Full Thoughts:

- ↝ I must never, ever skip my daily workout. That's the only way I'll succeed.
- ↝ I can't believe I ate that! I'm such a weakling.
- ↝ I could really be fit if I wasn't surrounded by all these temptations all the time!

Walking the Walk:
"I trust that good days will follow bad days, and that there will be more and more of the good ones as long as I stick to God's plan."

⌣ Walking for Other Reasons ⌣

"So, if you think you are standing firm, be careful that you don't fall! No temptation has seized you except what is common to man. And God is faithful; he will not let you be tempted beyond what you can bear. But when you are tempted, he will also provide a way out so that you can stand up under it."

1 Corinthians 10:12–13

If any man was ever tempted to relinquish his faith, it must have been the apostle Paul. On his missionary journeys, Paul endured incredible hardships, including hunger, cold, stonings, floggings, imprisonment, long days on the road, and even a shipwreck. Yet Paul resisted all temptations to curse his fate, trusting God to "provide a way out," as he says in this letter to the members of the Corinthian church.

As you establish your routine of healthy and rightful living, think about what tempts you to stray from this path. Certainly it is nothing "except what is common to man." Others are going through the same things you are. Anytime you feel like these temptations are threatening to overwhelm you, remind yourself that God will not let you be tempted beyond what you can bear.

Why allow you to be tempted at all? Well, why do we test schoolchildren? Why do we do strength tests on our limbs when recovering from an injury? To be sure they are ready for the next level, ready to meet the challenges that await them.

Remember that you are not expected to win every time or resist every minor temptation. Baseball players who get a hit once in every three tries are stars. Even the best NASCAR drivers win only a few races a year. What's important is that you succeed most of the time and keep striving. Part of God's reason for testing you is to make sure you are not one of those perfectionists who crumbles if the tiniest thing goes wrong. That kind of spirit isn't very successful serving others in the real world. Do your best to stick to your ideals, knowing that occasionally you may fall. God will give you what you need to keep going.

⌇ Activities ⌇

Try any of these activities as a way to minimize temptation's hold on you.

- *Keep a bowl of bite-size raw veggies within reach throughout the day. Carrots, celery, broccoli, and cauliflower are good choices. Munch on them frequently. The goal is to keep yourself in a half-full state, where food doesn't seem especially appealing. Temptation will never get a foothold! Raw vegetables are low in calories but high in fiber and water, so they fill you up without making you gain weight. No dips allowed! And no fruit or nuts, which can add up to hefty calorie counts pretty quickly.*
- *Anytime you are tempted to do something you shouldn't, go for a walk instead! Make it a nice brisk one that gets your heart rate up. Afterward, with those postworkout endorphins flowing through you, consider the temptation again and see if it holds the same appeal. Most likely it won't!*
- *Turn the temptation over to God. When something is tempting you away from your healthy lifestyle, don't fight it with willpower; instead, ask God what you should do. Listen to the answer, and do what He asks!*

⌇ Fit Facts ⌇

Temptation Likes Convenience

The easier it is to give in to temptation, the more you will do it. One study measured how many chocolate kisses secretaries ate in a day, depending on whether the chocolates were on their desks (visible and within reach), in a desk drawer (not visible but within reach), or across the room (visible but not within reach). On the average, secretaries ate nine chocolates per day when they were on the desk, six per day when they were in the desk drawer, and just three per day when they were across the room. If you want to avoid temptation, keep your temptations where they can't get your attention.

Portion Control

Your body's satiety sensors are not as well tuned as you might think. Many studies have shown that we eat more food if served larger portions. In one study, doubling a pasta entrée caused women to eat 120 extra calories—yet they didn't feel any more full, or eat any less during the rest of the day. To control your calorie intake, avoid the pitfalls of seconds, family serving dishes, and immense restaurant portions.

Wine Goes with Food

You've probably heard how drinking one glass of wine with your dinner can greatly reduce your risk of cardiovascular disease. It's true! But only if you have that glass with your meal, so that the alcohol is slowly absorbed into the blood and can counteract the glucose-spiking effect of the food. Drink on an empty stomach and you actually increase your blood pressure. Drink only one glass a day in any case; more than that increases your risk for many health problems.

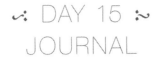
Tiptoeing Past Temptation

Affirmation

"Today I will do the best I can and not

punish myself for any mistakes I make."

Today's Walk

How Far? _____

Strength Training? _____

How'd It Go? _____

Notes

_____

_____

_____

A Witness for Fitness

Marilyn Allen and New Home Ministries
LaPlace, Louisiana

I have used Leslie's Walk Away the Pounds for Abs since 2002. I enjoy doing it so much that I sometimes do all three walks (one-mile, two-mile, and three-mile) in one session! Once while I was praying to the Lord with concerns about my own weight control, the Lord said, "Take your eyes off yourself and give women at church and in the community the knowledge that you have about nutrition and weight control." I started a class at church on April 3, 2005. Since then, the ladies have been steadily coming to get the information on fitness and health, and they have been enjoying the exercise sessions. I also enjoy every session of exercising with my beautiful sisters in Christ. I am more focused and conscious of what I need to do in order to stay fit and healthy. My energy level has increased and I am much closer to my target weight. The ladies call me their "motivator," but they motivate me and inspire me to continue doing what the Lord has called me to do. Our motto is from Philippians 4:13: "I can do all things through Christ who strengtheneth me." I thank God for Leslie and her walking buddies.

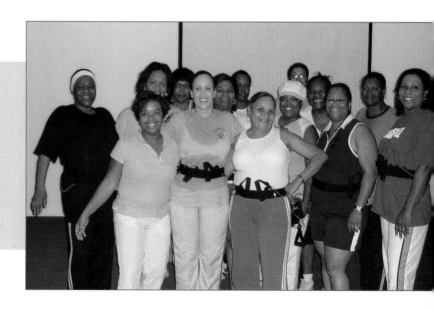

DAY 16

Playing with Time

We think of time passing at one steady, unchanging speed, but that isn't how we experience it. Time is amazingly elastic. Bits of time are like lollipops; they can be savored slowly or crunched up in a few bites. We usually learn the lesson pretty early in life that there is more pleasure to be had with lollipops by going the slow sucking route, but many of us never manage to apply this lesson to the rest of life. We crunch up life as fast as we can, hardly tasting anything because we're in such a rush to get on to the next lollipop, which will somehow be bigger and sweeter than the one we are currently holding.

There are a few problems with this. First, in the rush for the next lollipop, we tend to forget why we liked lollipops in the first place. Second, our physical health suffers when we go too fast for too long. And last, our spirits don't like all the rushing. Spirits are strong but slow. Getting them to unfold fully usually is a long process, requiring things that are in critical shortage in the modern world, such as quiet, contemplation, and peace.

On Day 12 of our thirty-day march toward wellness, we talked about slowing down and noticing what was going on around us. Now, on Day 16, we focus on stopping altogether and luxuriating in the "sacred now." Will this allow you to freeze time and stop aging? Not likely! But it may help you to understand that you have far, far more time than you thought you did—all the time in the world, in fact.

Playing with time this way does require some advance planning. Part of the reason we end up racing around is because of all the commitments we make: "Yes, I'll pick up the kids from soccer practice." "Yes, I'll meet you for a cup of coffee." "Yes, I'll cook dinner tonight." So if you are going to savor the moment today, make sure to keep your commitments to a minimum. A good day is when you have just enough to accomplish that you can do it at a sane pace.

You will find that when you slow down, enjoy the moment, and stop being eager for the next thing, you get at least as much accomplished as you did when you were racing around. How can this be? Don't ask me—I'm not a philosopher—but I'll bet it has to do with the fact that some of the things you *thought* you needed to do turned out not to be so vital after all. That's because you realized that you were not lacking anything; everything you needed, you had. Your impatience will be replaced by patience as you realize you are exactly where you're supposed to be.

As your patience and ease increase, the other thing that will happen to you is that your spirit will relax and settle in. You'll feel its divine presence much more often than you did when you were in five-alarm mode. And as you bask in that sacred glow, and your desire to prove yourself through end-less accomplishments wanes, you'll find that time has lost its power over you at last.

୰ Having Faith ୰

See if you recognize yourself in any of these un-faith-full thought patterns. Today, try to switch your inner dialogue so that your mind walks the walk along with your body.

Un-Faith-Full Thoughts:

- ୰ Let's speed this up so I can get on to something important.
- ୰ I need to stay busy because I don't like that feeling of emptiness when I stop.
- ୰ When I die, I want to have the most impressive obituary of all time.

Walking the Walk:

**"What I'm doing right now is exactly what I should be doing.
The past is done, and the future will take care of itself."**

❧ Walking for Other Reasons ❧

"There is a time for everything,
and a season for every activity under heaven:

a time to be born and a time to die,
a time to plant and a time to uproot,

a time to kill and a time to heal,
a time to tear down and a time to build,

a time to weep and a time to laugh,
a time to mourn and a time to dance,

a time to scatter stones and a time to gather them,
a time to embrace and a time to refrain,

a time to search and a time to give up,
a time to keep and a time to throw away,

a time to tear and a time to mend,
a time to be silent and a time to speak,

a time to love and a time to hate,
a time for war and a time for peace."
ECCLESIASTES 3:1–8

You are responsible for plenty of things in life, but thank goodness that time is not one of them! Time is a pretty huge responsibility, and God takes full charge of that. Knowing that you are off the hook, that everything is happening for a reason and that everything that needs to happen will do so in turn, frees you up to embrace the few things that are within your power. Notice how relaxed God is about time. He could speed up the universe so that His plan would unfold more quickly, but He doesn't. He is patient and knows that all things that happen are necessary things.

Do you get impatient for things to happen, or do you let each thing take its course? Do you read the end of a novel first, or do you enjoy the beginning, middle, and end in order? Think of your life as a novel or a movie. Each scene is important. There are no throwaway scenes. Since your life has far more meaning than any novel, every moment of it is impregnated with meaning. What changes in mental outlook can you make to stay aware of this with each passing moment?

༈ Activities ༈

Try any of these activities as a way to stretch the present moment to its most taffylike deliciousness.

- *Isolate yourself. Arrange to be stranded somewhere. Choose a day for yourself with no plans and have a friend drop you off at the library, or downtown, or at a park. Plan a pickup time for late in the day. In between, you have nothing to do but* be. *If you want to get really serious, plan to fly away for a weekend somewhere. Just make sure that your primary activity is nothing, beyond maybe a walk or two.*
- *Pick some yummy food that lasts a long, long time. (Yes, an occasional lollipop is okay!) As you savor it, do absolutely nothing else. Don't talk on the phone; don't wash the dishes; don't even enjoy the view. There is nothing but you and your lollipop. Don't rush through it; enjoy it at whatever pace it wants to be enjoyed. How does your experience of it change?*
- *Start a garden. Something about the nature of working with plants gives you a very different sense of time. Plants are awfully good at not rushing things. And few things make you lose track of time and obligations the way gardening does.*

∿ Fit Facts ∿

Supereggs

In the 1980s, eggs got an unfair reputation for being unhealthy, but they are actually nearly the perfect food—high in protein, vitamins, and good fat. Now some eggs are even closer to perfection. The company Eggland's Best feeds chickens a special vegetarian diet that helps them produce eggs that have 25 percent less saturated fat than regular eggs, 15 percent less cholesterol, and far more omega-3, vitamin E, and lutein, an antioxidant that boosts the immune system. The eggs cost about one dollar extra per dozen— the best dollar you'll ever invest in your health.

Walk to Beat Parkinson's

Add Parkinson's to the growing list of brain diseases prevented by exercise. Men who exercise regularly are 50 percent less likely to develop Parkinson's than are couch potatoes. And if the men start exercising in early adulthood, that likeliness drops an additional 10 percent.

Sleepy Nation

More than half of American women report not getting enough sleep and feeling sleep-deprived. Most of us need between seven and nine hours of sleep. Get less than that and the symptoms include poor performance on tests, weakened ability to store memories, sinking mood and possible depression, heightened stress, a slowed immune system, lower metabolism, and even weight gain. Skip a single night of sleep and your driving becomes as poor as a drunk driver's! Best ways to improve sleep: evening relaxation with yoga or meditation, quitting smoking, limiting alcohol and caffeine intake, a quiet and dark bedroom, and daily exercise at least three hours before bedtime.

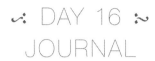

Playing with Time

Affirmation

"Today I will do one thing at a time.
I will give it my full attention and will enjoy it thoroughly."

Today's Walk

How Far? _____

Strength Training? _____

How'd It Go? _____

Notes

_____

_____

_____

That's Why They Call It *Faith*

At the beginning of this book, I wrote about the awesome power of faith. I said that I believe the single best way to get fit is with faith. I was talking about spiritual faith, but there are several definitions of faith, and they are all interconnected. Think about the everyday definition of *faith*. When you have faith in something, you trust that it's going to work out. You don't carefully calculate how it's going to work out, or pull the plug after a few days if things aren't going well. You just take a leap of faith and go for it!

It's no coincidence that many of America's greatest achievements were leaps of faith. Accomplishments from the Pilgrims' voyage to the Revolutionary War to the Wright Brothers' flight were not calculated gambles, but examples of setting a goal, acting on it, and trusting God. Most success— whether the goal is getting fit, getting promoted, or meeting the perfect mate—happens when we simply commit to the process and stop questioning things. Are you ready to make that leap?

You should be. It's not nearly as risky as you may have been led to believe, and your success may depend on it. A watched pot never boils, and a watched waistline rarely changes. Faith can help you get fit because it keeps you from "watching the pot" every day and worrying about whether progress is happening or not. And that's one thing you don't need to worry about. Progress is happening every day, around you as well as within you, but it can be hard to see it until you get some perspective.

In fact, a lot of progress can happen only when it's being ignored. We move toward our goals in fits and starts, not at a smooth and steady pace, and that herky-jerky rhythm is perfectly natural. If we fret over every detail and worry about failure right from the start, we put tremendous pressure on ourselves. Every down day or minor setback sets off alarms. On the other hand, when we trust the process and let things unfold at their own pace, we cultivate the peacefulness necessary for all growth and healing. A few people, such as professional athletes and actors, thrive when the spotlights are on them and the pressure is intense. Most of the rest of us do best when we are trusted to succeed and given the time to find our way and work things out.

Whatever you want in life, you must have faith that it will come your way. It won't happen without your participation—you still need to do your part—but one of the first prerequisites for making something happen is *believing* that it's going to happen. Then the pressure to perform is removed.

Think about something that you became really good at. It could be cooking or driving a car or using a computer. Chances are you weren't even aware that you were getting good at it. You just kept doing it, not paying attention to your progress or evaluating your performance every time. Suddenly, somebody complimented you on how you did it, and you said, "Yeah, I guess I am pretty good at this now." Without even realizing it, you'd mastered a task. That's how mastery happens—quietly, subconsciously, and with faith.

⌣ Having Faith ∾

See if you recognize yourself in any of these un-faith-full thought patterns. Today, try to switch your inner dialogue so that your mind walks the walk along with your body.

Un-Faith-Full Thoughts:

- ↴ This is crazy. I never should have started this in the first place.
- ↴ Things go wrong every chance they get. I need to be ready to abandon ship at the first sign of trouble.
- ↴ I need to stay on top of every detail and be in total control. I can't leave anything to chance.

Walking the Walk:
"Things are going fine."

⌁ Walking for Other Reasons ⌁

"Therefore I tell you, do not worry about your life, what you will eat or drink; or about your body, what you will wear. Is not life more important than food, and the body more important than clothes? Look at the birds of the air; they do not sow or reap or store away in barns, and yet your heavenly Father feeds them. Are you not much more valuable than they? Who of you by worrying can add a single hour to his life?
And why do you worry about clothes? See how the lilies of the field grow. They do not labor or spin. Yet I tell you that not even Solomon in all his splendor was dressed like one of these. If that is how God clothes the grass of the field, which is here today and tomorrow is thrown into the fire, will he not much more clothe you, O you of little faith? So do not worry, saying, 'What shall we eat?' or 'What shall we drink?' or 'What shall we wear?' For the pagans run after all these things, and your heavenly Father knows that you need them. But seek first his kingdom and his righteousness, and all these things will be given to you as well. Therefore do not worry about tomorrow, for tomorrow will worry about itself. Each day has enough trouble of its own."
MATTHEW 6:25–34

As an instrument of God, you know that He is going to keep you doing His work unless you manage to derail yourself somehow. Your best recipe for success is to stay out of your own way, so you don't trip yourself up. After all, in the long term, you're really the only one who can trip yourself up. And one of the best ways to do that is to lose faith and begin worrying about things you don't need to. Many people slip into a type of comforting anxiety, worrying about losing jobs when they have no reason to, or worrying about natural disasters, stock market crashes, food or oil shortages, or other things that are beyond their control and unlikely to affect them anyway. I say "comforting anxiety" because worrying about these distant issues is really a way of avoiding the things you can control: yourself, your commitments, and your life.

Having faith that God is going to take care of the big picture, and that you just have to do your small part, is essential to living a sane life. There's a reason they call it *faith*. It's because you have to trust that it's all working. If you start questioning every detail—"Why did God let me eat that bowl of ice cream?"—then you are going to exile yourself from the comfort and confidence that will bring you victory.

You are going to succeed. Never doubt it. Let tomorrow worry about itself. Today, walk forward with faith.

⸎ Activities ⸎

Try any of these activities as a way to escape doubt and embrace faith.

- *Cancel your newspaper subscription and turn off the evening news. For one thing, they simply make you worry about far-flung problems over which you have no control. For another, they relentlessly focus on the negative, because that is what brings in readers and viewers. The media will give you a distorted and gloomy view of life. Instead, focus on the firsthand information you get from friends, coworkers, and your own senses. Most of the time, your firsthand evidence will be that things are going pretty darn well.*
- *Read your Bible! If you ever have doubt that people have been able to overcome all manner of obstacles simply by having faith that God would see them through, you can read the stories of many such individuals in the Bible. If they triumphed through faith, you can, too.*
- *Many times in life, we face what feels like an insurmountable problem, but later when we look back at it, it seems minor. A twenty-foot cliff seems unclimbable, but once we discover that we can go around it, it is no big deal. We get locked into one way of solving a problem, not realizing that there are many other*

options. The next time you are faced with an "impossible" situation, remind yourself of the other "impossible" situations you faced in life, and how every single one of them worked out somehow (after all, you're still here, still living a normal life). View the situation from the perspective of faith, rather than getting locked in to the perspective of worry, and see if this opens up completely new ideas for you.

✌ Fit Facts ∿

Teens and Faith

Teens who value religion are three times less likely to drink alcohol, three times less likely to smoke, and four times less likely to use marijuana or other illegal drugs than are other teens.

Diabetes—the Lifestyle Disease

Most cases of diabetes can be attributed to our modern lifestyle: too much food, too little exercise. A daily walk and a sensible diet low in simple carbs and saturated fat can reduce your risk of diabetes by more than two-thirds!

Don't Stick with Nonstick

In recent years, people have become concerned that Teflon-coated non-stick cooking pans may release toxic gases when heated. The company that makes Teflon says that the pans would have to get to 680° F. before releasing gases, but if the idea of Teflon makes you nervous, consider switching to a different type of pan. Of the many available, good old cast-iron pans may be the best choice. They last forever, develop a virtually nonstick surface when seasoned properly, and have been used safely for centuries. Use a tablespoon of healthy oil (such as olive or canola) when cooking in cast iron to keep things nonsticky, or choose an enamel-lined cast-iron pan.

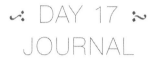

That's Why They Call It *Faith*

Affirmation

"Today I will do what is in my power to stay fit,
and everything else will take care of itself."

Today's Walk

How Far? _____

Strength Training? _____

How'd It Go? _____

Notes

_____

_____

_____

Trust

Whom do you trust? Your family, probably. A handful of friends, hopefully. A couple of coworkers, maybe. Are there others? Your boss? Your kids' friends? God? How about yourself? Trust is an incredibly powerful emotion, and it can make a lot of magical things possible, but it's an endangered species in the modern world. Trust is normally built on long-term relationships, on stable communities where people know one another and benefit from reciprocal kindness. Not everybody has that kind of long-term neighbors anymore.

But forget the neighbors; quite a few people out there no longer trust *themselves* to steer a just and healthy path through life. Are you one of those people? If so, today is the day to begin trusting yourself to get things right. You will. And that's because trust is not a passive quality; it's an active force that helps good things happen.

Think about what happens when you trust somebody. I mean *really* trust somebody, with something real. Say you're a manager of a business and you entrust a new employee with an important project. You can micromanage every decision, have the employee report to you every day, take all autonomy out of that employee's hands. What message are you sending? One that says, I don't think you can do this. You're going to screw up if I don't take charge. What you'll get in return is resentment and a poor performance (not to mention you'll be tying up your own time).

Instead, what if you say, "I trust you to do that. I know you'll do a really good job." You immediately empower the employee with your trust. When people are *expected* to do well, they usually do. They are uplifted by your confidence. (And, sure, you'll watch just carefully enough to make sure someone doesn't get in over her head.) Simply by trusting people, you have changed their perspective on themselves and on the world. That's pretty powerful!

When people know that you trust them, they are immediately inclined to trust you in turn. Trust engenders more trust! It can be a terrific force for healing and harmony in the world.

And what about yourself? You are currently engaged in an extremely important project: your health and happiness! You need to trust yourself to get the job done. Don't expect to fail! You may have been scarred by enough bad diet advice that you now expect to fail when you try once again to get fit, but that expectation of failure is exactly what's dooming you. Trust yourself to come through, because, remember, you aren't doing this alone. God is giving you everything you need to succeed, and you know that you can trust Him.

He's trusting you, too. He's not micromanaging. He's not pulling any strings. He's giving you all the love and fortitude you need, and trusting you to know what to do with it.

And you will.

⌣ Having Faith ∿

See if you recognize yourself in any of these un-faith-full thought patterns. Today, try to switch your inner dialogue so that your mind walks the walk along with your body.

Un-Faith-Full Thoughts:

- ∿ It's a dog-eat-dog world. I'm looking out for number one.
- ∿ If he's not part of my family, church, town, or country, then he can't be trusted.
- ∿ I've let myself down too many times. Why bother giving myself another chance?

"I trust in the goodness of the world, and in my own earnest intentions."

⌇ Walking for Other Reasons ⌇

*"May the God of hope fill you with all joy and peace
as you trust in him, so that you may overflow with
hope by the power of the Holy Spirit."*
ROMANS 15:13

Are you overflowing with hope? It sounds like a nice way to be, doesn't it? To get that feeling of abundant hope, you need to have a deep and abiding trust in God to get all the details worked out. Once you accept that, you can't help feel anything but hope, as well as joy, peace, and love.

This is a wonderful feeling that everybody should have, yet few do. What can you do to spread hope through the world? Whom can you bring into your circle of trust today, so that they, too, can overflow with hope?

⌇ Activities ⌇

Try any of these activities as a way to spread trust.

⚥ *Empower yourself to walk today by trusting yourself to do it. When you finish, congratulate yourself and assign yourself another accomplishment for the day. Say to yourself, I trust you to get it done. Then go right out and accomplish it. No pressure, no bargaining, and no punishment if you fail—just plain old trust. See how many things you can accomplish with it in one day.*

⚥ *Trust a total stranger with something important, like watching your belongings for a few minutes in a public place. See how this spontaneous act of faith changes your interaction. How does the other person respond in turn?*

❧ Try the classic trust activity: With a friend, take turns falling backward into each other's arms. It's corny, but it really does make for instant bonding!

⌣ Fit Facts ∾

The Trust Drug

Oxytocin is a natural hormone released by the body during times of bonding and trust. It reduces stress and increases feelings of clarity, contentment, and well-being. Breast-feeding mothers get huge surges of oxytocin in their blood, but you can also get it by snuggling or even just sharing something important. The connection works both ways: One study showed that after sniffing oxytocin, the subjects were twice as likely to trust a total stranger.

Good Cholesterol

You hear a lot about how bad cholesterol is, but what you don't hear is that there is a "good" cholesterol, too, and your body needs the good stuff just as much as it doesn't need the bad stuff. The good cholesterol, known as HDL, helps keep your arteries clean: Every extra point of HDL reduces your risk of death from heart attack by 2 percent. Best ways to raise it: Take daily walks; drink one glass of wine per day; eat lots of foods high in good fat, such as olive oil, fish, and nuts; lose weight; and, of course, stop smoking.

Get That Pressure Down

We all know high blood pressure is bad. How bad? It increases your risk of heart attack seven times! Even slightly elevated blood pressure (higher than 120/80) increases your risk three times. That's why it's so important to get regular exercise and eat a balanced diet.

Trust

Affirmation

"Today I will apply no pressure to myself to succeed.
I trust that it will happen naturally."

Today's Walk

How Far? _____

Strength Training? _____

How'd It Go? _____

Notes

_____

_____

_____

A Witness for Fitness

The Go-Go Grannies: Pat Pogose and Linda Willis
McHenry, Illinois, and Richmond, Illinois

We are two proud grandmas who want to say that "Les" is more, and we'll tell you why.

Pat: *I gained weight in middle age and eventually weighed 256 pounds. Then I got leukemia. After extensive treatment, I was so weak. Leukemia left me in a sorry state physically and mentally. I still needed to lose weight, but I had to do something to get stronger. Walking was the answer.*

Linda: *I was fifty-five when my friend Pat's health crisis gave me an epiphany: My own health deserved a closer look. I started out walking with Pat to help her recover and achieve better health, but I knew in the process I would improve my overall health and vigor, too. At the beginning of our walking program, we proceeded slowly, gently, and gradually. Very short walks on a regular basis turned into longer ones. When we were*

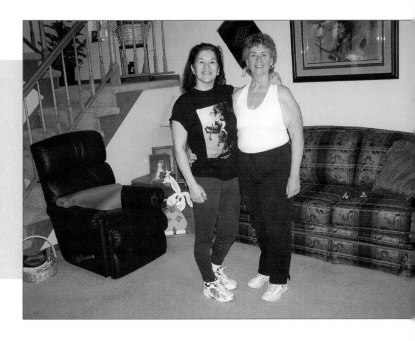

already walking two-mile stretches, we decided we needed a boost to our regimen. Enter Leslie's walking program—the springboard and core of our program. Pat got the videos, we added them to our walking regimen, and voilà! We were on our way!

Pat: *I was fifty-six when I started with Leslie. I was out to get a healthy mind and body after being so sick, and I have. In addition to losing eighty-six pounds, I feel much better about myself and have an improved attitude overall, I do more daily activities without tiring, and I have many more clothing choices—and I actually look good in them! In the shower one day, I noticed my triceps was tightening up and there was less fat. Another day on a walk in the park, I noticed my shadow went in at the waist! Wow, another red-letter day! My daughter, Bridget, says, "Since my mom has started exercising, she is a much happier and stronger person. So much so that she has inspired me to get on the bandwagon, too!" Bridget uses Leslie's videos, too, now.*

Linda: *My daughter, Julia, also joins us occasionally and has commented on how much more flexible and energized I have become. This is great, especially since I work with her in her residential cleaning business. I have the endurance it takes to handle the rigors of the job. My fitness also ensures continued assignments in my other part-time job—as a senior artist's model. Our life goal is to keep moving and feeling good well into old age. Our good health is also a gift of insurance to our kids; the longer we can care for ourselves, the less of a burden we will be to them. Now I feel fearless about trying fun new ways to exercise that get me playing with my kids and grandkids. I've even taken up snowboarding, cross-country skiing, and Rollerblading! Most valuable to keeping our commitment to health is Leslie's brand of inspirational, enthusiastic encouragement. For almost three years now, her voice has been a record in our heads, bolstering our self-esteem. Yes, you can do anything without killing yourself. As Leslie says, "You can't do it wrong!" Give her an "Alleluia!"*

Don't Just Talk the Talk

In the basements of America lies the discarded evidence of past noncommitments to exercise. Stationary bikes gathering dust. Dumbbells and yoga mats and elliptical trainers. All these items were purchased with good intentions and were embraced, however briefly. But they didn't last. Why not? Because the commitment came from the outside. Somebody bought the right gear, embraced the newest "breakthrough," and hoped that if they talked the talk long and loudly enough, they'd walk the walk, too.

There's nothing wrong with talking the talk. It can help us stay focused on our goals. But it needs to come from the inside out. Ideally, we talk the talk because we are walking the walk all day every day, and it is such an authentic part of who we are that we can't *not* talk about it.

Think of the people you know who have a deep and abiding passion. It could be for anything, from staying fit to saving the rain forest. You know they mean it not from what they say but from the way they act, the way they *live* their passion every day. If nobody else on the planet were watching, they'd be doing the very same thing. *That's* devotion!

Does your devotion to health and fitness come from the inside or the outside? Every now and then, it's worth checking yourself and making sure that you aren't just going through the motions. Even a walking program that begins out of genuine desire to improve can slip over time, and without you ever realizing it, you are talking the talk, while inside you are looking for any excuse to jump ship.

So how about it? It's been nearly three weeks since you began reading this book and walking with me. Are you still there? Still my daily companion?

And are you doing it for me, or for yourself? Still 100 percent devoted? That's the spirit! Nothing feels better than being the authentic you.

↶ Having Faith ↷

See if you recognize yourself in any of these un-faith-full thought patterns. Today, try to switch your inner dialogue so that your mind walks the walk along with your body.

Un-Faith-Full Thoughts:

- ↷ If I volunteer for that organization, it'll look really good on my résumé.
- ↷ I think I'll wait to do my walk today until my friend comes over for lunch, so she can catch me doing it.
- ↷ I have to exercise to keep my looks.

Walking the Walk:

"I am devoted to walking. It's part of my worship."

↶ Walking for Other Reasons ↷

"And when you pray, do not be like the hypocrites, for they love to pray standing in the synagogues and on the street corners to be seen by men. I tell you the truth, they have received their reward in full. But when you pray, go into your room, close the door and pray to your Father, who is unseen. Then your Father, who sees what is done in secret, will reward you. And when you pray, do not keep on babbling like pagans, for they think they will be heard because of their many words. Do not be like them, for your Father knows what you need before you ask him."

MATTHEW 6:5–8

Since before Matthew wrote those words, people have been pointing out that the truly faithful are often the quiet ones. Not the ones chanting their prayers the loudest in church or on street corners, but the ones saying them alone in their rooms with fervor. The ones who make it *personal*.

When you commit to anything and make it personal, you have no one to fool. Excellence is the usual result of this. You can't fool yourself, and you can't fool God. You can't even show off, because no one knows what is expected of you except *you*. We sometimes think that excellence happens when the challenge is great, the stakes are high, the world is watching, and an individual rises to the occasion, like a singer on *American Idol* or a quarterback in the Super Bowl, but I admire the kind of excellence that happens every day when no one is watching and when the rewards are entirely personal. That's the excellence of devotion, the purest form of love. Good things come from that.

If you ever find yourself slipping into a laundry-list prayer—"Let me walk two miles today and help me get over this flu, and while you're at it, there was that raffle I entered yesterday . . ."—remember Matthew's words: "your Father knows what you need before you ask him." We don't pray to get favors granted. We pray to check in. When your authentic self reports for duty, everything else takes care of itself.

✌ Activities ◡

Try any of these activities as a way to test your faith and fitness resolve.

- *Put yourself in this scenario: Your family is out of town for the week, your friends are busy, and I can't see through the TV screen. No one will know whether you walk today or not. Will you still do it? Why?*
- *Take a one-week vow of silence when it comes to discussing your walking program. You don't bring it up to others, and if they mention it, you just shrug and change the subject. You simply* do *the walks for their own sake, without reinforcement, positive or negative, from others. After a week, do you feel more enthusiastic about walking, or less? If less, you might have been talking the talk more than you needed.*

❧ *Do something beautiful that no one will ever know about, or that you will never get credit for. Leave an anonymous present for a stranger. Draw a beautiful picture, then burn it. Build a sand castle on an empty beach, even though you know the tide will level it in an hour. In that act of creating beauty for its own sake is the spark of pure devotion. Try to capture that feeling and hold it inside you when you walk.*

∿ Fit Facts ∿

Calcium + Tryptophan = Zzzzzzz

Studies show that the nutrients calcium and tryptophan help induce sleep. (Calcium also builds strong bones and reduces PMS symptoms by 50 percent.) A glass of skim milk (calcium) and a banana (tryptophan) make an ideal bedtime snack.

Where Your Sugar Lurks

Forget dessert; the number-one source of sugar in the American diet is soft drinks. Not surprisingly, those drinks are one of the leading contributors to diabetes. Women who drink sugary sodas more than once per day have nearly twice the risk of diabetes as women who drink sodas less than once per month. Drinking fruit punch also contributes to diabetes risk, while consuming natural fruit juice doesn't.

Cinnamon for Diabetes?

The next breakthrough diabetes medicine may be good old-fashioned cinnamon! USDA researchers have found antioxidant compounds in cinnamon that enhance insulin's ability to metabolize sugar twentyfold! This helps explain why volunteers who ate half a teaspoon of cinnamon every day for forty days reduced their glucose levels by 20 percent.

Don't Just Talk the Talk

Affirmation

"Today I walk in silence for the beauty of walking."

Today's Walk

How Far? _____

Strength Training? _____

How'd It Go? _____

Notes

_____

_____

_____

Perseverance and Discipline

What keeps people going? What is the difference between Lance Armstrong and, well, the rest of us? And how do we become more like Lance? The answer may be surprisingly simple.

You may be tempted to say, "Come on, Leslie! Lance Armstrong is a fitness machine. I've read that he can carry more oxygen in his blood and utilize it more efficiently than almost any human on the planet. He's no model for me!"

It's true that very few of us can perform at Lance's level. But those physical abilities are not what got Lance up and on his bike every day, year after year, in blistering Texas heat and bone-chilling French rain. It's not what made him survive cancer and get through chemotherapy treatments that would have driven almost anyone into retirement but that, in his case, helped him not just to get on a bike again but to come back *better* than before, and win the Tour de France an astonishing seven times. No, we can't aspire to match Lance on a bike, but we can definitely use him as a model of perseverance and discipline for our own lives.

So what *does* keep Lance Armstrong going? It isn't simply a matter of winning. He's lost a lot of races. When he first came back from cancer and started training again, when winning the Tour de France was nothing but a pipe dream, he crashed and burned a lot. Not everyone realizes this, but he actually quit cycling for a while. In the middle of a race in France, he simply pulled over to the side of the road and quit. Why put up with the misery? He had nothing to prove. So he went home to Austin, Texas, and played a lot of golf and ate a lot of Tex-Mex.

And he felt terrible about himself.

Ring any bells? We've all quit things, convinced ourselves that it really didn't matter to us if we persevered, when deep down it did. You can tell yourself that staying in shape is not a big factor for you, yet you know how high your spirits were when you were making progress and how down in the dumps you felt when you weren't. The same has been true for Lance, though his highs have been a lot higher and his lows a lot lower than most of ours.

Eventually, Lance Armstrong got back on his bike, knowing that to be truly living we need to keep moving forward. "The old routines and habits," he said, "like shaving in the morning with a purpose, a job to go to, and a wife to love and a child to raise, these are the threads that tie your days together and that give them the pattern deserving of the term 'a life.' "

Then came discipline. Once he was back to riding every day, he kept his goal in sight—winning the Tour de France—and simply did what he needed to do each day to achieve that goal. That's all you need to do each day, too—maintain the discipline to move closer to your goal. You don't have to get there right away; you just need to maintain momentum. Be disciplined about it, not because there is any inherent virtue in discipline, but because *you* will like yourself better at the end of the day. And you will have a longer, healthier, and more joyful life, too.

During that 1999 Tour de France, as Lance broke away from the pack in the French Alps, climbing peaks and shattering records, he realized what it was that had lured him back to his calling and that allowed him to ride effortlessly up brutal mountains: "the sheer exultation of being alive."

And that's something we all can identify with.

↶ Having Faith ↷

See if you recognize yourself in any of these un-faith-full thought patterns. Today, try to switch your inner dialogue so that your mind walks the walk along with your body.

Un-Faith-Full Thoughts:

- What's the point in getting fit? I'll just go backward eventually.
- I think I'll slack off today. I don't want this that badly.
- Another setback. People who succeed at this never have setbacks. I just don't cut it.

Walking the Walk:
"Perseverance? Discipline? What's so hard about that?"

∾ Walking for Other Reasons ∾

"Consider it pure joy, my brothers, whenever you face trials of many kinds, because you know that the testing of your faith develops perseverance. Perseverance must finish its work so that you may be mature and complete, not lacking anything. If any of you lacks wisdom, he should ask God, who gives generously to all without finding fault, and it will be given to him. But when he asks, he must believe and not doubt, because he who doubts is like a wave of the sea, blown and tossed by the wind."

JAMES 1:2—6

"Why me?" That's the first thing we are all tempted to ask when something goes wrong. Why us? How can life be so unfair? It's a natural reaction—we've been trained since childhood to think that good behavior automatically triggers rewards—but the result is that such self-pitying thoughts kill our drive and momentum. We can get sucked into a spiral of hopelessness.

Yet we've all overcome trials of many kinds in our lives. Not just overcome them but used what we learned in those tests to grow stronger and wiser. You would not be the capable person you are now without those tests. You wouldn't trade those valuable experiences, so why feel any differently about the new trials awaiting you?

Nothing will serve you better in life than to "consider it pure joy" when you get to confront a challenge of any kind. You know full well that God is going to keep you on your toes by throwing you plenty of curveballs, yet you also know that He isn't going to throw at you more than you can handle. This includes challenges to your faith, illnesses and other challenges to your health, and many other tests. When the next curveball comes along, thank God for keeping you sharp, then knock it out of the park.

∽ Activities ∾

Try any of these activities as a way to keep yourself strong and focused.

- *The next time something goes wrong, act ridiculously enthusiastic about it. Thank God, grin like an idiot, and rub your hands together in eager anticipation of tackling the problem. Do it when others are around so that they look at you like you're insane. You won't really feel so positive about things, but you'll enjoy the humor of acting a bit crazy, and when you do come down to reality, you'll still be at a place of optimism and engagement—much better than the defeatist mentality you could have adopted.*
- *Anytime you feel your resolve weakening, project into the future. If you are considering a large piece of chocolate cake, weigh the momentary pleasure of eating it versus the uncomfortable stuffed feeling afterward and the poor sense of well-being for hours thereafter. If you're thinking of skipping your walk or skipping church, think about how good you feel after doing those things. A big part of maturation is learning to ignore impulses and act based on how we are going to feel later, and for the rest of our lives.*
- *Act under orders—your orders. Like a private in the army, once you get an order, you must carry it out; there's no debating whether or not you should do it. Once you give yourself an order, whether it's to walk six times a week or abstain from sweets—you have to stick to it. This takes all the mental wrestling out of the equation. You were told to do it, and you're going to do it. That's what discipline is.*

⌣ Fit Facts ∾

You Have the Power

In a *Consumer Reports* survey of 32,000 people who attempted diets, the big winners were the ones who acted on their own to change their exercise and dietary routines. Of the most successful weight losers—those who lost an average of thirty-seven pounds and kept it off for five years—83 percent did it without following an official program or diet or joining any group. Only 12 percent used meal replacements such as meal shakes, and just 6 percent used diet pills or other supplements.

Walk Diets Beat Food Diets Every Time

In the same *Consumer Reports* survey, 80 percent of successful weight losers who tried exercising at least three times a week listed it as their number-one weight-loss strategy. A solid 40 percent also used the strategy of adding small bits of exercise (such as choosing the stairs over the elevator) to their daily routines, and 29 percent used some sort of weight lifting to increase their calorie burn.

Vivaldi for Your Brain

In an Emory University study, volunteers who listened to Vivaldi's *The Four Seasons* while exercising performed twice as well on a vocabulary test after exercising as the volunteers who didn't listen to music while exercising. *The Four Seasons* is known for its ability to stimulate the brain, but other types of up-tempo music should work also.

Perseverance and Discipline

Affirmation

"I have a spirit that is dedicated
to being fully and exuberantly alive."

Today's Walk

How Far? _____

Strength Training? _____

How'd It Go? _____

Notes

_____

_____

_____

Habits

You have reached a very special day in the Walking the Walk program. Performance experts know that a period of twenty-one days is the typical time it takes to develop a new habit. There are both mental and physical reasons for this, but they all have to do with the way your body constantly adjusts itself to your needs. Your body continually tries to get better at whatever is asked of it, concentrating its resources where they are needed. It's a great survival mechanism! If you carry heavy objects every day (or do strength training), that stress on your muscles is your body's signal to build larger muscles, so you'll perform better the next day. (You've experienced the flip side of this if you've ever broken an arm or leg and been in a cast. After just a couple of weeks, those muscles are *gone.* Use it or lose it.) If you challenge yourself with crossword puzzles every day, then your body focuses its energy on creating new connections between neurons, so your brain can process more words more quickly the next time. If you walk a couple of miles every day, your body creates more enzymes for turning food and oxygen into fuel, so you can walk farther on the same amount of energy.

Over a single day, these changes are almost unnoticeable. But with time, they become quite real, and the twenty-one-day period is the key. At that point, your body has made enough physical adjustments that the new task will start to come easily to you. More important, it has laid down the mental pathways in your brain so that you *anticipate* the new behavior. Think about how you get hungry just before mealtimes. That's because your body has an excellent internal clock, so if it has learned to expect food at a certain time of day, it starts making gastric juices in your stomach and pumping saliva into your mouth, ready to digest that food as efficiently as possible. Your body is good at anticipating lots of things, from waking you up just as your alarm is about to go off to triggering an absolute craving for a cup of coffee in mid-afternoon.

Habits are physical and mental behaviors that have made well-worn paths in our brains. Once established, they happen almost unconsciously; in fact, it takes terrific concentration to *break* them. This cuts both ways. If you crave nicotine after a meal and the result is a smoking habit, that has terrible health consequences. But if your habit is walking first thing when you wake every morning, and you've done it so long that your shoes practically lace themselves when you swing your feet out of bed, then that habit is going to serve you well.

The secret to long-term health is to develop as many healthy habits as possible. Habits are like personal trainers who show up at your door every day and make you stick to the program. You don't have to make the mental effort to force yourself to do it; you just obey the personal trainers. And, as I said, a period of twenty-one days is the turning point. For twenty days, you've been making yourself do your new activity. Every day it's been getting a little easier, and now, on Day 21, the weight swings to the other side of the seesaw. Your body and brain are anticipating the new activity, and it would actually take more conscious effort to *stop* the activity than to keep doing it.

So today is a cause for celebration. If you have been faithfully walking the walk with me for twenty days, then after today you are home free! Barring injury or earthquake or some other major hurdle, you are going to keep walking away the pounds and walking your spirit into a state of grace. It's part of you now! Part of your day, part of your worship, part of your character. Congratulations on one terrific habit!

∿ Having Faith ∿

See if you recognize yourself in any of these un-faith-full thought patterns. Today, try to switch your inner dialogue so that your mind walks the walk along with your body.

Un-Faith-Full Thoughts:

- ༄ I can skip my walk whenever I want. It doesn't matter as long as I do it now and then.
- ༄ I'm just not one of those people with enough drive to do something regularly.
- ༄ I'm trapped in my bad habits and there's no way out.

Walking the Walk:

**"I make my habits, and then they make me.
I can choose my habits and will choose carefully."**

⌣ Walking for Other Reasons ∿

*"I will extol the Lord at all times;
his praise will always be on my lips.*

*My soul will boast in the Lord;
let the afflicted hear and rejoice.*

*Glorify the Lord with me;
let us exalt his name together.*

*I sought the Lord, and he answered me;
he delivered me from all my fears.*

*Those who look to him are radiant;
their faces are never covered with shame.*

*This poor man called, and the Lord heard him;
he saved him out of all his troubles."*

PSALM 34:1–6

In this chapter, we've talked about the benefits of developing good physical habits, but what's the very best habit of all? To extol the Lord at all times. No matter whether things seem like they are going well or not, whether you feel like the odds are stacked against you or like you can do no wrong, you still want to have His praise on your lips. It's a habit, like any other. In this case, the habit will keep you from going to the dark places of resentment and self-pity. Resentment can be the worst of all habits. If you resent others for their success, or the ease of their lives, or for getting in the way of *your* success, you may start to feel that life isn't fair, or that happiness and fulfillment just aren't your lot in life. This habit can become a knee-jerk reaction to any downturns in your day, and it can become a *very* tough one to break.

But happiness and fulfillment are up to you. You make them or you don't; it's not up to life to provide them. Develop the habit of glorifying the Lord, of thanking him for your great fortune, and you will find that joy was there all along, waiting for you to discover it. And the joyful habit is one that will serve you well throughout your days.

⌇ Activities ⌇

Try any of these activities as a way to use your habits to your best advantage.

- ❦ *Make a list of all your habits—all the things that you do more or less automatically each day. Now mark them as good habits or bad habits. The good ones will take care of themselves, but how did the bad ones start? What can you do to reverse them? Pick one and try.*
- ❦ *Create a new good habit in your life—flossing, for example. For the next twenty-one days, it won't come easily, so do whatever you need to do to force the habit into place. Put reminders up for yourself, leave packages of floss all over the house, and don't allow yourself to watch TV until you've flossed. After twenty-one days, see if the habit is locked in. If so, pick another good behavior and start again! You are now one of those self-empowered people!*
- ❦ *Make a habit of thanking God. You may do this from time to time when something wonderful happens—"That truck didn't hit me, thank God!"—but that*

doesn't make it a habit. Thank God habitually for all the little goodnesses in your day, the rain and the sun and a steaming cup of coffee at 7:00 AM, and notice how there is no time to dwell on the less good parts—because it's all good in one way or another!

⤳ Fit Facts ⤳

Take Religion to Heart

The Jackson Heart Study, a study of more than five thousand African-Americans, found that those who actively participated in religious activity had considerably lower blood pressure than those who did not participate.

Exercise Beats Zoloft

In a study of 156 clinically depressed people, thirty minutes of vigorous exercise three times per week was more effective at lifting depression than the antidepressant Zoloft. It's more effective at slimming your waistline, too!

Four SuperMini Lattes to Go!

Researchers have found that caffeine is far more effective at keeping you alert if taken in small doses over an extended period of time. About two ounces of coffee every hour will help you pull an all-nighter more successfully than a sixteen-ounce coffee drunk all at once. Sleep, of course, might be the best option of all!

Habits

Affirmation

"Daily exercise is a part of me now. My cells *crave* it!"

Today's Walk

How Far? _____

Strength Training? _____

How'd It Go? _____

Notes

_____

_____

_____

A Witness for Fitness

Elisa Lochridge
Tigard, Oregon

I am thirty-seven years old. I was heavy most of my childhood and young adulthood. I managed to lose weight for a while, but then I gained twenty pounds before I got pregnant with my third child. I experienced complications and was ordered to bed for most of the pregnancy, so, needless to say, I gained a lot of weight. The week before I had my son, I weighed 219 and was asked by a clerk in a store if I was having triplets. When I said no, she said, "Please tell me twins." When I said no again, she asked why I was so fat. I was so discouraged! After giving birth, I went down to 190, but that was still the highest I had ever been when not pregnant.

A friend of mine told me about Walk Away the Pounds. *I had tried other expensive workouts in the past and could not work the gadgets, or the steps were too confusing, but I started the two-mile walk and was amazed at how easy the steps were. Even*

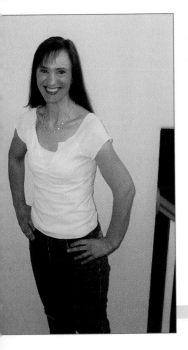

though I am very uncoordinated, I could keep up and wasn't tripping over my own feet. I started doing it a few times a week. I gradually worked up to doing it five to six times per week. Then I graduated to the three-mile walk, and after a few months, I was doing the three-mile walk eight times per week!

I am now at 121 pounds and feel the healthiest I have ever felt. I am also encouraged and reminded during workouts that the ability and strength to move are blessings that come from God. Many times when I wanted to give up, I just remembered that and thanked the Lord that I do have the ability to move my body. I just want to say, Thanks, Leslie, for coming up with such a great program, and thank you, Lord, for Your strength in helping me lose the weight and become healthier, and thanks for Your faith in me to see me through.

Prayer and Meditation

I'm sure you will agree with me that prayer is an important part of worship, but agreeing on the kind of prayer is another matter. There are as many ways of praying as there are people to pray, and they can all be done with sincerity. What I want to focus on today is a style of prayer that can be particularly effective with your fitness goals: meditation.

When some people think of meditation, they picture bald Buddhists in orange robes on top of Himalayan peaks closing their eyes and chanting for hours. But meditation can be any practice that focuses the mind on one particular thought or image, and it's been an essential devotional method for Christian monks for a millennium. Normally, our minds flit around like moths. Try concentrating on anything, and within a few minutes you are humming "Achy Breaky Heart" instead! Like anything else, mental concentration takes practice, and today most of us aren't very practiced. But intense mental concentration is the key to opening a path of communication between your spirit and God's. You can fire off your usual prayers over dinner or in church, and that's about equivalent to sending E-mails to your senator: It counts, but don't expect any personal answers. Prayerful meditation, however, is like discovering a direct hot line; be prepared for some intense communication! Some of the greatest moments of life can be these times when your mind is so perfectly tuned to God that you are overcome by feelings of fulfillment and belonging.

As you can imagine, these glorious feelings are payback enough for the time invested in meditation, but there are plenty of additional paybacks, as well. Meditation keeps the body healthy by reducing stress and lowering blood pressure (see today's Fit Facts for additional benefits). You come out of meditation with improved concentration and clarity of purpose; it makes you a better, less distracted worker, parent, and performer.

It makes you a better walker, too. That practice of keeping the mind on task for long stretches spills over into your regular day. You get better at focusing on what needs to be done and recognizing what is just a distraction, and better at sticking to something once you start it.

Now, here's the really crazy part. Walking can be meditation! You don't need the orange robe and Himalayan peak; just some sweats and sneaks and the enclosed DVD, and away you go! Music and repetitive physical movements are two classic tools for generating a higher state of awareness, so walking to the beat of the accompanying spirituals is the fast track to a state of mental intensity that we could call "the Devotion Hot Line." Use it as needed to refresh your spirit and recharge your body.

⌣: Having Faith :~

See if you recognize yourself in any of these un-faith-full thought patterns. Today, try to switch your inner dialogue so that your mind walks the walk along with your body.

Un-Faith-Full Thoughts:
- ⌇ God already knows how I feel. There's no need to actually form the thoughts in my mind.
- ⌇ Meditation? Isn't that what New Age Yuppies do?
- ⌇ Prayer should only be done in a pew.

Walking the Walk:
**"When my mind is free from distraction and focused on prayer,
I get that daily dose of spirit that keeps me strong."**

～ Walking for Other Reasons ～

*"Do not conform any longer to the pattern of this world,
but be transformed by the renewing of your mind.
Then you will be able to test and approve what God's will is—
his good, pleasing and perfect will."*
ROMANS 12:2

We all know how the world and its constant mundane needs can get us down. Day after day, the wear and tear of just getting everything done can certainly steal our joy if we let it. But rather than let ourselves conform to these patterns, we need to get renewed periodically by a fresh jolt of spirit. Where do we look for such a jolt? To meditation, the whole purpose of which is to renew our minds.

Re-new, "to make new again": That sounds pretty good to me. A new mind, uncluttered by worries or grocery lists or old hurts—that's what you get through prayer and meditation. It's like taking a bath in the cleansing waters of the Holy Spirit. When you don't get those baths periodically, your spirit gets slowly caked with the grime of daily life and all the compromises made to get through the day and keep everyone happy. Eventually, it becomes difficult even to recognize your spirit under all the grime. And that's the danger—that you'll forget about your spirit and its needs entirely.

Make sure to renew your mind regularly, whether at church or by meditating at home. While you're at it, do you know others who could use a little mental and spiritual rejuvenation? Invite them to join you in a refreshing round of prayerful meditation or spiritual walking and get those spirits scrubbed clean and shiny again!

◡∴ Activities ∴◡

Try any of these activities as a way to improve your ability to use the mind's "spiritual Internet."

- *Join a meditation group. No matter what the goal of the group is, you will learn great techniques for focusing the mind and controlling your thoughts, which will help you in numerous areas of life, including work, sports, prayer, art, and stress-reduction.*

- *Use a prayer as a mantra while you walk. A mantra is a repeated phrase or a series of syllables that meditators use to free their minds from mundane distractions. You could pick any short prayer that you know by heart, or you could come up with a sentence that is meaningful to you and your goals. Repeat the words over and over and over as you walk. It may feel a little silly at first, but at some point the repetitiveness of it will turn the words into a background rhythm, allowing the mind to float away into the realm of real creativity and spiritual connection.*

- *Try a little solitude. Most people find that meditation is most effective when they are completely alone. When you aren't interacting with others, or even thinking about interacting, your mind becomes free and receptive to Spirit. Good bets for solitude: wilderness areas, city parks, private offices, or even, in a pinch, the bathtub.*

◡∴ Fit Facts ∴◡

Meditators Have More Brains

You already know that prayer and meditation can reduce stress and heighten feelings of relaxation, but new research shows it can make you smarter, too. People who had meditated for years had significantly more brain cells in the areas governing memory and attentiveness than did people who never meditated.

Take the Edge Off

In a study of chronic headache sufferers, 72 percent reported moderate or great reduction of their headaches after learning to meditate. And 91 percent of anxiety sufferers reported significantly reduced anxiety after learning to meditate.

A Prayer a Day Keeps the Doctor Away

A study found that regular prayer reduces visits to doctors and other health-care professionals by an amazing 50 percent.

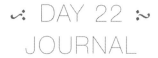

Prayer and Meditation

Affirmation

"Today I will make the effort to set the world aside for a few minutes and let my mind enter the realm of Spirit."

Today's Walk

How Far? _____

Strength Training? _____

How'd It Go? _____

Notes

_____

_____

_____

The Power of Music

If you think about it, food and drink are far from the only things we "feed" our bodies. Every second or so, we breathe air—along with whatever microscopic hitchhikers are riding in the air—into our lungs, where the oxygen is transferred into our blood. Light constantly enters our eyes, registers on our retinas, and causes electrical signals to be sent to the brain. Similarly, sounds enter our ears, are converted to electrical signals, and travel on to the brain, where they cause physical changes in neurons.

None of this is news, but what is news are the many studies showing that the quality of the sounds that surround us have a profound effect on our moods, energy, and even our health. The right sounds can make us perform better, resist illness, and think happier thoughts. Yet we pay amazingly little attention to controlling our sonic environment. It's time we start thinking of sound as a nutrient every bit as important as vitamin C or calcium.

If sound is a nutrient, then the ultrapotent multivitamin form of it is music. You know instinctively what an incredible impact music can have on you. It can fire you up and make you feel like you can take on the world, or it can chill you out and make you feel as peaceful and relaxed as a purring cat.

For proof of the power of music to change your thinking and even the way your body feels, look no further than the enclosed DVD—or your nearest gospel church. It's all about rhythm. The rhythms of music entrain with your brain waves, literally altering your thought patterns. When you hear the word *entrain*, think *train*; get your brain on that train, and let the music do the work while your brain gets a free ride to the land of high energy, of spiritual glow, or wherever that particular musical train is heading.

But that's the rub, because there are sonic trains heading to all kinds of places, some good, some bad. Are you feeding your ear sonic junk food or wholesome, uplifting sustenance? It's not just a matter of the music in your home and car. Environmental noise, such as the noise from traffic or airplanes, can be terrible for your health. It raises blood pressure and the number of stress hormones in your body. It causes hearing loss as well as sleep disruption, and the latter leads to everything from poor concentration to depression and increased risk of accidents. Constant noise also inhibits a student's ability to learn.

Starting today, take a noise audit of your daily life. Are there places where noise is reducing your quality of life? Are there places where the right music could improve your mood and performance? What can you do to start making sound work for you, not against you?

◡: Having Faith :◡

See if you recognize yourself in any of these un-faith-full thought patterns. Today, try to switch your inner dialogue so that your mind walks the walk along with your body.

Un-Faith-Full Thoughts:

- I like that blast of angry energy I get from rap or heavy-metal music.
- Noise and sounds have no effect on my mental state. I block it all out.
- I just can't get inspired to exercise. I'd rather sit here and listen to my iPod instead.

Walking the Walk:
"I don't eat junk food and I don't listen to junk sound."

∿ Walking for Other Reasons ∿

"Shout for joy to the Lord, all the earth,
burst into jubilant song with music;

make music to the Lord with the harp,
with the harp and the sound of singing,

with trumpets and the blast of the ram's horn—
shout for joy before the Lord, the King.

Let the sea resound, and everything in it,
the world, and all who live in it.

Let the rivers clap their hands,
Let the mountains sing together for joy;
let them sing before the Lord,
for he comes to judge the earth.
He will judge the world in righteousness
and the peoples with equity."
PSALM 98:4–9

Music and spirituality go together like two hands. For thousands of years, people have used music to celebrate the glory of the Lord. Singing is many people's favorite part of church, and no wonder; it's never easier to feel the presence of the Holy Spirit than when your whole chest is vibrating with the power of a favorite hymn. The entire universe is made of cycles and vibrations and rhythms, and music lets us feel how we are a part of that spiritual energy.

It also makes the perfect bridge for connecting spirituality and fitness.

Physical exercise is also all about rhythm—the pump of your heart and lungs, the steady balance of your steps, the flow of air in and out. When you're moving in sync with the right music, and you feel your soul connected by that musical string right to God, you just *know* you're doing exactly what you should be at that moment. Since the very first exercise class that I led, at St. Joseph the Worker Church in New Castle, Pennsylvania, I have ended all my classes with inspirational music, allowing God to do his most amazing work on the heart of each person. Just try not feeling empowered, calm, and connected when that double whammy of music and postworkout rush hits you!

As you walk to your favorite spiritual music and you feel the power, shout for joy before the Lord! With your system charged by Spirit, you have the power to walk as far and as long as you desire. You're not just listening to the music; you *are* the music.

⌣ Activities ∾

Try any of these activities as a way to make the most of the music and sounds in your life.

- *Try a sonic experiment. Walk with me as you usually do, letting the music on the DVD uplift you. On your next walk (same day if you're feeling energetic), play the DVD, hit the mute button, and put on some real downbeat music instead. How was your energy and mood affected? Are there other places in your life where inappropriate music could be holding you back?*
- *Visit a church known for its gospel music. You'll feel the Spirit like never before! If you like the surge of positive energy this gives you, keep visiting. Or take some of the music home on CD and play it whenever you need to change the mood.*
- *Kick noise pollution out of your life! If you hear significant traffic or office noise where you work, consider wearing headphones while playing music that helps you focus. If your kids blast music that sends your stress levels through the roof, buy them a nice set of headphones. If Jet Skis, leaf blowers, or car alarms disturb your neighborhood's peace, get together with other citizens and educate your neighbors on the very real damage these devices are causing.*

༝ Fit Facts ༘

Music—the New Aspirin

People with chronic pain (from arthritis and other conditions) who listened to relaxing music reduced their incidence of pain by 21 percent and depression by 25 percent.

Music—the New Antibiotic

Specially designed stress-reduction music, which uses soothing rhythms to lower heart rate and blood pressure, played to volunteers for fifteen minutes increased their immune-system function by 55 percent, while rock and New Age music had no impact.

Music—the New Personal Trainer

In a survey of college students, 97 percent said they believed music helped their aerobic performance, especially by making the experience more enjoyable for them and motivating them to keep doing it.

The Power of Music

Affirmation

"Today I will fill my soul with powerful,
energetic, and uplifting music!"

Today's Walk

How Far? _____

Strength Training? _____

How'd It Go? _____

Notes

_____

_____

_____

Cleaning Your House
of Bad Beliefs

Who are you? If asked that, how would you answer? Most of us form our self-image surprisingly early in life, and often it doesn't change much after that. We get a variety of labels attached to us, and more often than not, we take those labels to heart. "I'm unathletic." "I'm an underachiever." "I have a weight issue." "I'll never be rich." It's amazing the inaccurate, unnecessary baggage we carry around in our heads just because of something someone once said to us! Generally, these beliefs are based on very flimsy evidence. They certainly wouldn't stand up in court!

Here's a different way of looking at the question. Imagine that someone said to you, "You are an amazing person. You're such an achiever, I've got no doubt you'll succeed in your goal of creating a healthy and fulfilling life." Would your first reaction be to think, You know, that's absolutely true! or would you immediately start discounting the statement in your head and thinking of reasons why it isn't true? If the latter, then you've got a severe case of the bad-belief blues, because we've spent the past twenty-three days learning that you *already* have all the tools you need to achieve lasting physical and spiritual health!

But this isn't just a question of your self-image. What other bad beliefs do you hold? Do you believe people are generally kind or that they're cruel? Do you believe you are lucky or unlucky? Do you believe life is meaningless or that it's a vital spiritual journey? Do you believe good things happen most of the time or that life is a series of catastrophes that you need to be prepared for?

The thing about all these questions is that there are no proven answers to any of them. If there were, then there wouldn't be so much disagreement about what the "right" answers are! You may say, "Well, Leslie, I've been around, and I've had a lot of experience that has led me to be a pessimist." But somebody else will come along and have just the opposite point of view, based on their life experience.

It comes down to choice. Optimism is a choice. Happiness is a choice. Trust is a choice. Our beliefs are choices we make, and those choices have a strong influence on how we live our lives, how we interact with others, and what experiences we have.

I'm a "glass is half-full" kind of person. I tend to see the bright side of things, and that tendency has served me well. I started my fitness career teaching aerobics in church basements for donations. I sure didn't have a business plan, I just believed that others would be as passionate about exercise as I was—and they were. Years later, I took a big risk going on QVC for the first time with my workout videos. I just believed people would respond well—and they did, beyond my wildest dreams. Now I'm trusting that people will be interested in hearing my beliefs that physical and spiritual health are intimately connected. I don't know how things will work out, but I've sure got a good feeling about it!

How about you? Are your beliefs helping you or hindering you? What can you do today to begin fostering a belief system that will make your life as enjoyable, successful, and loving as possible?

∿ Having Faith ∿

See if you recognize yourself in any of these un-faith-full thought patterns. Today, try to switch your inner dialogue so that your mind walks the walk along with your body.

- ∾ I'd like to be happy, but I doubt that I ever will. It's not my style.
- ∾ My life isn't very meaningful, but I'd rather make a lot of money than do something I love and be poor.
- ∾ This country's going downhill and there's no way to save it.

Walking the Walk:

**"I control my present, and I make my own future.
I will be exactly who I want to be."**

∾ Walking for Other Reasons ∾

*"Whatever you do, work at it with all your heart,
as working for the Lord, not for men."*
COLOSSIANS 3:23

You may think that the prospect of consciously changing your belief system sounds impossible, and it's true, it's difficult to change things that are deeply ingrained in us. That's why it can be best to take an indirect route. After all, the beliefs that hamper your joy by making you feel angry or frustrated or disconnected probably stem from some direct assumptions about the world that you learned early on. If you learned to focus on making money or always winning or even distrusting other people, it can be hard to break free into a state of joy and fulfillment.

So go about it the other way around. "Whatever you do, work at it with all your heart, as working for the Lord, not for men." Embrace that notion, and suddenly everything begins to change. When you throw your heart into something, when you do it for a reason bigger than yourself, you'll discover joys in your daily work that you never suspected. You'll encounter other people reaching out with their hearts to join you in sacred work. And your assumptions about the nature of other people, and the nature of life, will change without your even realizing it. You'll learn that the joy and integrity you thought nearly impossible to find were inside you all along.

༈ Activities ༈

Try any of these activities as a way to shift your belief system toward a more rewarding worldview.

- *Pretend you have to describe yourself to someone who doesn't know you. "What's she like?" they ask. Now tell them. List as many things as you can think of to describe what you're like. Then read over the list. Does this sound like someone you'd enjoy knowing? Now make a list describing the qualities of the ideal person you'd like to be. What are the differences in the two lists, and what is preventing you from being that ideal person? Why not start acting like that ideal person today?*
- *Count your blessings. Each day, record three things that went well. In a study of ways to increase our happiness, this method was one of the most effective and long-lasting. Another effective method is to make a "gratitude visit" by writing a letter of thanks to someone who has helped you and delivering it in person.*
- *Actively get in touch with a friend or family member each day. Studies show that the strongest indicator of a rewarding and optimistic life is having strong social ties.*

༈ Fit Facts ༈

What America Believes

Religion has a positive influence in the world: 80 percent

Americans are less moral and honest than they were fifty years ago: 80 percent

Young people have less sense of right and wrong than they did fifty years ago: 81 percent

Children are more likely to grow into moral adults if raised in religious households: 60 percent

What *Doesn't* Make You Happy?

Studies show that the following factors have little or no bearing on happiness: age (older people may actually be slightly happier), income, weather, IQ, marriage, and education.

What Makes You Happy?

When asked "What one thing in life has brought you the greatest happiness?" people's top answers were:

Children or grandchildren: 35 percent

Family: 17 percent

Faith or religion: 11 percent

Spouse: 9 percent

Cleaning Your House of Bad Beliefs

Affirmation

"Today I will act with integrity toward myself
and will reach out to others with love and kindness."

Today's Walk

How Far? _____

Strength Training? _____

How'd It Go? _____

Notes

_____

_____

_____

A Witness for Fitness

Walk-by-Faith
Pittsburgh, Pennsylvania

God spoke Walk-by-Faith into existence. Our purpose is to promote healthier life-styles so that the church and community may be spiritually uplifted. Through the in-spiration of God, a group of women started meeting on Saturdays under Kaufmann's Clock to walk the perimeter of downtown Pittsburgh. On Sunday mornings before church service, we would walk around Schenley Park. That winter, Leslie's videos were presented to us so that we could keep walking indoors through the winter season. Now we meet three times a week at the church to walk and stretch. The response has been overwhelming. Through God and all the supports He has provided from the community, the group has grown to fifty-two participants. It consists of infants, toddlers, young adults, the middle-aged, and the elderly, all walking together and changing our lives in the process. Sister Diane has lost 120 pounds and says, "Through Walk-by-Faith, I am staying more active, whether it is walking outside or enjoying Leslie's Walk the Walk series inside." Sister Debbie has diabetes, but she says, "The walking helps to keep my blood-sugar level down and I am truly grateful to God for not having to take medicine now for three to four years." We want to give God all the praise, honor, and glory for the group's success. "To God be the glory for the things He hath done."

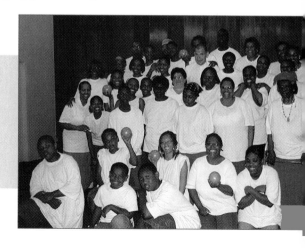

Outfoxing Stress

You can't hide from stress. It will find you. It will find you at home, on the job, during the commute, and pretty much anywhere else. Stress is a part of daily life in America. We have to accept that. But what we shouldn't accept is the impact of stress: the damage it does to our bodies, minds, and spirits. If you've been saddled with way too much stress for way too long, today is the day to start doing something about it.

You may be tempted to say, "What's the big deal? Stress is a regular part of life. You just get used to it after awhile." But that's the danger. A little bit of stress is normal, and you can get used to more and more stress, but while you come to expect incredible stress and even think of it as normal, your body is silently suffering under the load. You may think stress is normal, and you may also think being frazzled at the end of the day is normal, being unable to sleep is normal, feeling anxious and depressed is normal, and having deteriorating health is normal. None of these is normal, and none is an acceptable part of your life. Stress is the element to focus on to begin turning things around.

Stress can mean any number of different things. Illnesses or physically demanding jobs can cause physical stresses on your body. Family tension, hectic jobs, and hazardous driving cause mental stress. But stress is stress; whatever the cause, the effect is the same: increased stress hormones in your body.

Your body is no dummy. It makes those stress hormones (primarily adrenaline and cortisol) for a reason. They make you perform better. The stress hormones make your heart beat faster, lungs work faster, brain think faster. Your senses sharpen and your muscles take in extra energy. You are more alert, quicker to respond, and faster on your feet. You perform at your very best, which is what those stress hormones are trying to do. A challenge has come up—you need to meet a deadline or avoid a deer in the road or ace a job interview—and your body is trying to help you out. Great. If stress was a rare occurrence, this would be a perfect system.

But stress isn't rare, and that's the problem. In our modern lives, we encounter constant stressors, so our bodies are constantly releasing fresh supplies of stress hormones, keeping us on high alert all the time. And when we are full of stress hormones, we can't relax. That's deadly, because a number of important things happen only when we relax.

You can't get something for nothing, and the increased performance you get from stress is a trade-off. The extra energy comes by shutting down bodily tasks that aren't essential at that moment. The systems that get shut down are the ones involved in long-term health: the immune system, digestive system, and reproductive system. Your memory gets spotty and your cells stop repairing themselves. Brain chemicals associated with happiness aren't maintained.

We think of relaxation and sleep as activities where nothing much is going on, but that's when your body accomplishes most of its maintenance. Under chronic stress, you don't relax and you don't sleep, so maintenance doesn't happen. Your body breaks down, just like a car that's driven hard and long without oil changes or tune-ups. Aging accelerates. Rates of cancer, cardiovascular disease, and gastrointestinal disease climb. Women have more trouble getting pregnant.

Scared yet? Don't be, because while you can't hide from stress, you can outfox it. Learning how to reduce stress in your life and how to deal with the stuff you can't avoid can make all the difference. There are no revelations here. You know what you need to do; it's just a matter of raising it to the top of your priority list. If you are overburdened at work, start initiating or suggesting some changes so you can get more help; your health and happiness depend on it, so it's not something you can keep putting off. If your family or personal life are the big sources of stress for you, see what changes you can instigate there—do you really need to be participating in all your current activities? As for the stress you can't avoid, see today's suggestions for activities that will help you process that stress and get it out of your body as quickly as possible.

Start tackling your stress problem today. Your family will thank you. Your friends will thank you. Your body will thank you. And your spirit will thank you.

✌ Having Faith ✌

See if you recognize yourself in any of these un-faith-full thought patterns. Today, try to switch your inner dialogue so that your mind walks the walk along with your body.

Un-Faith-Full Thoughts:

- Bring on the stress! I thrive on going a mile a minute, on doing five things at once, and I hate the boredom of slowing things down. I'd rather live twice as fast and half as long.
- I feel so alone. I have so many worries and no one to help me. I just feel like giving up.
- I'm so behind! If I cancel my social activities, drink another cup of coffee, and pull an all-nighter, maybe I can get caught up.

Walking the Walk:

"Stress comes and goes, but if I keep exercising and relaxing and trusting God's plan, I'll stay on an even keel and everything will take care of itself."

✌ Walking for Other Reasons ✌

*"Trouble and distress have come upon me,
but your commands are my delight."*
PSALM 119:143

From time to time, trouble and distress are going to find you. That's life. Your challenge is not to avoid them entirely—impossible—but to find solace when you are distressed and to keep going. The first casualties of stress are your sleep, your joy, and your spirit, but you can save all three of those by remembering your delight in God when times get tough.

Part of the danger of stress is the spiral effect: We start out worrying about some job-related stress, and that keeps us up at night, so then we begin worrying about not sleeping enough, and then we worry that high stress is going to make us sick, and on and on, with our worrying spiraling out of control.

The real root of all this worrying is the belief that things are not going to be okay. When you feel that train of thought coming on, switch tracks to God instead. Think on Him and remind yourself that things are going to be okay, that the big picture is still in place. A few blips in the road will not change that. Rather than let stress come crashing down on your stability, you can build on your spiritual foundation and structure a life that sheds stress like rain off a new roof.

↶ Activities ↷

Try any of these activities as a way to reduce your stress load.

  ⭘ *Save your walks for the evening. The most common time for people to walk with me is in the morning, before life gets too crazy. That works great for some people, but if you find that you come home from work every day dragging a wagonload of stress, you might want to walk it off then. Exercise is the best stress reliever known; it gives your body a way to burn off all that edgy, adrenaline-enhanced energy and gets you back to equilibrium so that you can have a peaceful evening and a good night's sleep.*

  ⭘ *Cut your caffeine intake. Coffee and tea can be great comforts, and having a cup or two a day does no harm, but any type of caffeine raises your stress hormones. If you feel jittery or have trouble sleeping, stop drinking caffeine after lunch. If you still have trouble, consider cutting out your morning caffeine, too.*

  ⭘ *Relax. Praying, socializing with friends, playing games, taking baths, doing yoga or meditation, and even curling up with a good book all serve to reduce stress hormones in your body.*

⌁ Fit Facts ⌁

Sleep Away the Pounds

The Nurses' Health Study, which tracked the health and habits of 68,000 women for sixteen years, found that women who slept five hours a night were 32 percent more likely to gain significant weight (thirty-three pounds or more) over the course of the study than were women who slept seven hours a night. The shocker? The women who slept seven hours a night actually ate slightly *more* than the women who slept five hours a night. Both groups got similar amounts of exercise. How could this be? Sleep deprivation may prevent your body from burning calories efficiently. Whatever the case, it's one more reason to sleep well, eat well, and walk well.

Stress at Work

Stress affects you indirectly in more ways than you know. About 80 percent of employees feel stress on the job, 29 percent have yelled at a co-worker, 24 percent have cried due to job stress, and 19 percent have quit a job due to the stress. Accidents on the job are stress-related about 70 percent of the time. And Americans work longer hours and have more job stress than people in any other country. The health problems due to all this stress are incalculable.

Stay Sharp

Not all stress is bad. A little daily stress in the form of challenges and activity keeps you sharp. That's why people who retire suffer, on average, an 8 percent increase in illness, an 11 percent drop in mental health, and a 23 percent increase in difficulty performing daily tasks within six years of retiring. The solution? Keep working. People of the same ages who kept working at least part-time didn't suffer the same problems.

Outfoxing Stress

Affirmation

"Today I will give it my all, do what I can,
and not worry about what I can't do."

Today's Walk

How Far? _____

Strength Training? _____

How'd It Go? _____

Notes

_____

_____

_____

Getting Whole Again

Do you ever feel like a collection of disjointed computer programs, rather than a whole person? There's the Hard Worker you, the Stern Parent you, the Loyal Friend you, the Good Christian you, and on and on—and none of these yous seem to be connected. You just turn on whichever program you need to get through that part of the day.

We sometimes compartmentalize the various aspects of our lives in order to deal with them efficiently. How could we not? It works, and it keeps things going. But once we've broken our self into small, efficient pieces, often something gets lost when we try to put the pieces back together. That something is what makes you unique. Call it your soul. For it to thrive, all the aspects of you and your life need to be functioning in perfect harmony so that thought, feeling, and spirit can flow through you.

If you are having trouble sensing your sacred self, today is the day to start mending your inner fractures. Remember that you are not merely the sum of your abilities and experience and character traits. You are so much more. You are not random; you were made for a purpose. You just *know* when you are on your life's path and when you aren't. It feels so good to be in accord with your nature, and it just doesn't feel right to be at odds with it.

Sometimes you have some part of your life that you just don't feel quite right about. It might be a job that you can't put your heart and soul into, or a friendship where you feel like you're pretending to be someone you're not. You try to convince yourself that your discomfort will go away, but deep down you know better.

Today, ask yourself if there are any parts of your life about which you aren't being honest with yourself. What can you do to adjust those parts so that everything works together as a seamless whole? So that everything you do contributes to your purpose?

How will you know when you're whole again? You'll know because every aspect of your life will support the others, rather than draining them. If your job is out of balance with your life and purpose, you come home from work so drained that you can't enjoy your family, so that part suffers, too. If you are physically out of shape, that exhaustion and illness can detract from your career, your friendships, and virtually every other facet of your life. But when you are whole, your high physical energy lets you sail through the workday, which leaves you energized in the evening for quality family time, which leaves you feeling so blessed that your spirit can't help but soar, which leaves you sleeping peacefully and being ready the next morning for a fun workout. Everything gets easier!

You should feel filled with purpose on a daily basis. That doesn't mean things won't be hard sometimes, or that you won't suffer bad luck and the occasional setback. But it does mean that even during hard times, you won't waver from your commitments and won't have to question what you're doing. You'll know you're being you, through and through, and you'll love yourself for it. And that's the *whole* truth!

⌣ Having Faith ⌣

See if you recognize yourself in any of these un-faith-full thought patterns. Today, try to switch your inner dialogue so that your mind walks the walk along with your body.

Un-Faith-Full Thoughts:
- I don't feel good about doing this, but it's easier to do it than to make a big deal out of it.
- I'm not into soul-searching. I just let the chips fall where they may.
- Life doesn't have any deep meaning. I just try to keep myself happy.

"I know that living a life of purpose requires me to take care of myself, outside and in, and to keep making sure I'm doing what I really believe in."

⌣∴ Walking for Other Reasons ∿

". . . We do not know what we ought to pray for, but the Spirit himself intercedes for us with groans that words cannot express. And he who searches our hearts knows the mind of the Spirit, because the Spirit intercedes for the saints in accordance with God's will. And we know that in all things God works for the good of those who love him, who have been called according to his purpose."

ROMANS 8:26–28

In this chapter we've discussed making sure that all parts of your life and personality are devoted to furthering your life's purpose. This is important, but don't worry too much about figuring out what your life's purpose is. You will know it when it happens. You may even have been doing it for some time before you realize how right it is for you. In any case, don't fret it. If your heart is open and full of love, the Spirit will intercede and steer you true. Let your love for God guide you, and you can trust that you are always living according to His purpose.

⌣∴ Activities ∿

Try any of these activities as a way to reestablish your sense of your sacred self.

❧ *What makes you unique? What makes you different from anyone else on the planet? Carve out an hour for yourself to do nothing but reflect on this question and jot down some answers. Remember, this isn't about what other people would say makes you unique. No one knows you like you do. List the things that you know in your heart make you special.*

❧ *Nothing makes you feel like one seamless person quite as much as exercise. With your heart and legs working, your brain humming with endorphins, and your skin prickly with sweat, you can* feel *the way your body and mind are perfectly integrated. Use your next walk as a time to reflect on how good it feels to have your whole self working in tandem. What can you do in your life to get this wonderful feeling more often?*

❧ *Envision an ideal week in your life. Not a vacation week, but an ideal yet regular and realistic week. List all the things that get accomplished in that week, and all the things you do for fun. Include some romance and laughter and physical activity. Now compare your ideal week to your actual week. What are the factors in it that feel "wrong," that prevent you from achieving a good week? Isolate one or two that are within your control, and make the effort to change them next week.*

⸙ Fit Facts ⸙

The Thrifty Gene

Life can be unfair, and one howling example of that unfairness is the so-called thrifty gene, a gene more common in overweight people, which can put a cruel twist on the energy balance equation. People who possess the thrifty gene can be as much as 15 percent more efficient at getting calories from their food—meaning they have to eat 15 percent fewer calories, or burn 15 percent more, to maintain the same weight as someone who doesn't have the thrifty gene. But even if your body is "thrifty," you can still lose weight—you just have to go that extra mile!

The Microbe Connection

The cutting edge of obesity research involves studying the microbes that thrive in the human digestive system. You have plenty of these microbes (by weight, your body is more microbe than it is human being!) and they accomplish a lot of beneficial tasks for your body, one of which is assisting with digestion. The proportion of different types of microbes in your gut affects how easily you store fat. In a few years, you may be able to take dietary supplements that change the balance of microbes in your gut and make it harder for you to absorb fat!

Help for Migraines

Migraine headaches are three times more common in women than in men, and they can certainly ruin both physical and spiritual health, making it impossible to drive, exercise, think, or do anything other than lie in a darkened room and wait for relief. But recent breakthroughs have made migraine treatment more effective than ever. Medicines are now available that prevent most migraines. And certain things that were once believed to trigger migraines, such as alcohol, chocolate, and cheese, have been shown to have no connection. However, estrogen levels, which fluctuate monthly, do have a connection. If you suffer from migraines, or other frequent headaches (most of which are undiagnosed migraines), ask your doctor about the new treatments.

Getting Whole Again

Affirmation

"I am a whole, sacred person.
There is no one like me on Earth,
and I'm going to have a blast while I'm here!"

Today's Walk

How Far? _____

Strength Training? _____

How'd It Go? _____

Notes

_____

_____

_____

DAY 27

Forgiveness

There's a famous saying: Revenge is a dish best served cold. It means that you shouldn't try to get revenge on your enemies right away, when they're expecting it, but should wait until everyone but you has forgotten, so it can be a surprise. But the saying should really be this: Revenge is a dish served by cold stiffs. That's because the stress of harboring resentment for years will do in people before they ever get to the revenge!

In the real world, forgiveness beats revenge every time. Revenge, resentment, grudges, obsession with old injustices—what do these have to do with you and where you are right now in your life? Responding to old insults only counts on some imaginary cosmic scorecard of justice that no one cares about.

Don't let resentment simmer in you. Forget whether you have a right to feel resentment toward someone or not; the only thing that matters is that the resentment is going to cause *you* pain and stress. Letting it go and practicing forgiveness, whether the person is deserving or undeserving, can be a powerful tonic for finding peace within yourself.

This can be a tough concept to accept. We are so programmed to think about rewards for good behavior and punishments for bad that we naturally try to extend that to everyone we interact with. "Why should I forgive *him?*" you ask. "What he did was totally wrong!" He did the crime, and now he's got to do the time, right? Except (a) the punishment—your eternal anger—is probably something he'll hardly notice, and (b) who is the main person who is going to suffer from all that anger? You are!

That's a key to forgiveness—the realization that the only person suffering from all these hard feelings you have is you. Forgive the deserving because they deserve it and the undeserving because *you* deserve it! Don't "throw the baby out with the bathwater" by making yourself feel miserable just because somebody else did something you didn't like. Don't let anger eat you up.

This doesn't mean you forget about what somebody did, or will let them do it again, or approve of the action in any way. But it does mean that you release the hurt and don't keep it bottled up inside, where it can continue to hurt you.

And what about when *you* do something you don't like? Do you berate yourself about it endlessly? Why? What do you hope to gain? Try thinking about it from the other side. You're committing these thirty days to improving your physical and spiritual fitness. What attitude toward yourself will best help you achieve that goal? That's all that matters, and we all know what the answer is: forgiveness, love, and support. Who cares if you skipped your walk one day or cheated on your diet? You're not in *The Sopranos,* and it's not about crime and punishment. It's about peace and joy.

⌁ Having Faith ∿

See if you recognize yourself in any of these un-faith-full thought patterns. Today, try to switch your inner dialogue so that your mind walks the walk along with your body.

Un-Faith-Full Thoughts:

- ↷ I never forget an insult. I keep careful mental track of who has done me favors and who hasn't.
- ↷ I'll never forgive what she did to me. I think about it all the time. Someday I will have justice.
- ↷ I'll never forgive myself for all the stupid things I've done. At this point, I'm guilty until proven innocent.

Walking the Walk:

"Everybody has their imperfections, including me, and I bear nobody any malice. My love extends to all humankind—myself included!"

✌ Walking for Other Reasons ☙

". . . Clothe yourselves with compassion, kindness, humility, gentleness and patience. Bear with each other and forgive whatever grievances you may have against one another. Forgive as the Lord forgave you. And over all these virtues put on love, which binds them all together in perfect unity."
COLOSSIANS 3:12–14

There are deeper reasons for forgiveness than the fact that it will make your life and health better. Forgiveness is among the most fundamental of Christian virtues, and it's central to many of Christ's teachings, from "turning the other cheek" to the parable of the prodigal son. When somebody who has messed up comes back, you don't give them their just deserts; you celebrate! Consider Matthew 18:21–22. When Peter asked Jesus, "Lord, how many times shall I forgive my brother when he sins against me? Up to seven times?" Jesus' reply was, "I tell you, not seven times, but seventy-seven times." After all, the Lord forgave all mankind for all of our sins; the least you can do is forgive a few people (or yourself) for some of theirs.

A good thing to keep in mind is that morality should not operate on a sliding scale. Everybody gets the same treatment, because it's not about what they've done or haven't done; it's about how you want to live your life. And you know that you want to live a life of love, clothed in "compassion, kindness, humility, gentleness and patience." Embrace this mission and you will be amazed at how simple it makes decisions and reactions you used to think were difficult.

⌁ Activities ⌁

Try any of these activities as a way to forget old scores and achieve inner peace.

- *Make a list of all the people or institutions that you hold some sort of grudge toward. Write each one a letter explaining that you forgive them, that you understand the situation was complicated and that "things happen," and that you wish them well in the future. Now here's the key part:* **Don't send the letters!** *If you do, it will just be interpreted as lording the moral high ground over them. You need to mean the letters when you write them, but then throw them away and simply be left with the peace of real forgiveness.*

- *Do something nice for someone who doesn't deserve it—especially someone who would never expect you to do something nice for them. See how your act changes the relationship to an unfamiliar, unpredictable, and usually more fulfilling one.*

- *Forgive yourself. There's no one you are more likely to blame for old screwups, and no one who needs your forgiveness more. Write down on scraps of paper the things from your past that still make you wince, then burn them one by one. As you do, feel that old issue disappear once and for all. Instead, love yourself for doing the best you can every day.*

⌁ Fit Facts ⌁

Repent Your Resenting

Resentment and unforgiveness produce classic stress symptoms in the body: raised levels of adrenaline and cortisol, which result in hypertension, cardiovascular disease, reduced immune response, and increased depression, paranoia, and anxiety. People who were coached in forgiveness training, however, were able to alleviate all these symptoms.

No Melatonin Miracle

Three-quarters of Americans have trouble sleeping at least a night or two every week, and more and more of them are turning to melatonin, a natural hormone that helps regulate sleep cycles—melatonin levels rise at night and go down during the day. But a major new study has found that melatonin is no miracle. If you need to sleep during the day—because of jet lag or working a night shift, for example—melatonin supplements work great, because they give you the level of melatonin, and sleepiness, your body would normally have at night. But if you suffer from insomnia, melatonin can't help. You already have all the melatonin you need for sleeping, so the problem lies elsewhere. Cutting down on caffeine and exercising at least three hours before bedtime are good places to start.

Anger Kills

In a Michigan study, women with increased anger had twice the mortality rate of women with little anger. It didn't matter whether the women suppressed or vented the anger—the idea that letting it out is worse than bottling it up is a myth; demonstrating anger just led to more anger later. The worst health risks were associated with cases in which women were angry about situations over which they had little or no control. If you have hope of controlling and eventually remedying a situation, you suffer fewer health risks from the anxiety associated with it.

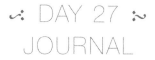

JOURNAL

Forgiveness

Affirmation

"I begin today with a clean slate.
I hold nothing but love for myself and everyone I meet,
and I will act in all of our best interests."

Today's Walk

How Far? _____

Strength Training? _____

How'd It Go? _____

Notes

_____

_____

_____

A Witness for Fitness

Roxanne Wenzel
Sun Prairie, Wisconsin

I started my journey to a healthier me in September 2004. At age forty-five, I weighed over 250 pounds and wore a size twenty-four W. I was on medication for high blood pressure and was extremely out of shape. I often had trouble taking stairs and regularly ran out of breath after expending small amounts of energy.

I first started using Leslie's program after watching my sister tone and firm herself from a size twelve to a size eight. At first, I could barely make one mile and would almost fall over during the stretching. I persevered and made it to two-, three-, and then four-mile walks. I used the Stretchie, weighted balls, and ab belt to add resistance and tone my muscles. During this time, I also changed my eating habits to include healthy foods and plenty of water.

In just a few months, my blood pressure was under control and I was able to stop my

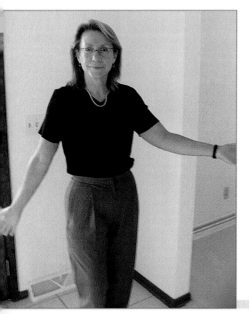

medication. The more weight I lost, the better I felt and the more I enjoyed doing Leslie's workouts. I started doing a different routine every day and added her shortcuts and other firming routines. I had never been a fan of exercise, but now I work out with Leslie every day. I am not exaggerating when I say that I feel better today than I have in my entire life.

In one year, I lost 100 pounds and have lost 116 pounds in total. Even more impressive is how much lean muscle I have gained during my transformation. I am happy, healthy, full of energy, and able to do so much more in my life. Everyone comments how I always have a smile on my face. Thank you, Leslie, for giving me a much better quality of life!

Doing It for Them

I've got a surprise for you today. It's Day 28 of your thirty-day commitment, but it's already time to declare victory. You've succeeded! If you've made it this far, you are home free. You have been acting like a physically and spiritually fit person for four weeks, and when we act like something long enough, we become it.

Does that mean you get to slack off these last three days? Far from it. Because, as you well know, it's not about just you. It hasn't been about you from the beginning—in fact, that was one of your initial keys to success. By taking the focus off yourself and committing to physical health as part of your faith, you've been able to achieve more than you might have if you'd felt you were all on your own.

Now it's time to pass the favor on—time to do it for them. Who are "they"? That's going to be different for each of us. Maybe you have children who can benefit from the lesson that their physical fitness and sense of self-worth are intricately linked. Maybe you have friends or siblings who need a helping hand to get off the couch. Maybe you want to start a walking group at your church. We all have others in our lives who can use our help—even if we don't realize it.

Sometimes this help can be active, as when you approach a friend and say, "Hey, I know you're feeling down in the dumps and your self-esteem is gone. I recognize it because I've been there, too. And getting yourself back on track is easier than you can imagine. Let me show you what worked for me." Sometimes, all you need to do is model good behavior and others will follow. It can be much more effective to be a model than a drill sergeant, especially if you have kids. Kids will resist you if you use threats to make them turn off the video games and play outside, make them eat their vegetables instead of junk food, and so on—especially if they see that you are guilty of the same vices you are banning for them. But if all around them, you and other adults lead healthy, active lives and spiritually fulfilled ones, and enjoy it, then the lessons will sink in by osmosis. You may not think so, but everything is being taken in by those quickly developing brains.

Some of my moments of deepest joy have been at the baptisms of my three children. I feel that my greatest responsibility in this life is to raise three more faith-filled people. I believe that guiding children to a life that serves God is a parent's real job; everything else will work out from there!

Make no mistake about it: Kids need you and others like you. Many kids don't have good role models, and many factors in society are encouraging them to move less and eat more. Obesity has never been higher among kids and adults. The rate of diabetes has never been higher. We need all the good role models out there we can get. Which is why, when you are out Walking the Walk, you are doing it for us all.

If you've got the wrong attitude, it can feel like a burden to think that you need to be a role model for the next generation in all that you do. But that's the social contract. Think about all the help you received from the previous generation as you were growing up. More important, if you have the right attitude (which I know you will), it can feel amazingly good to realize that you are now in the position of helping others. What a rush! How far you've come. The ultimate testament to your newfound success is the fact that others might look to you and think, She's got all that energy and spirit. I wonder if I could ever be like that? Show them that they can!

⌣ Having Faith ⌣

See if you recognize yourself in any of these un-faith-full thought patterns. Today, try to switch your inner dialogue so that your mind walks the walk along with your body.

- ✂ I don't have time for anybody else. My work and my workouts are all I can deal with.
- ✂ These kids aren't grateful enough for what I'm doing.
- ✂ I've struggled so much to achieve the success I have. Who am I to give advice or be a role model?

Walking the Walk:

**"Just as I am part of God's plan, so is everyone else.
I've been so blessed in life, and I know one of the greatest
blessings is the chance to pass that on."**

⌇ Walking for Other Reasons ∿

*". . . Always be prepared to give an answer to everyone who
asks you to give the reason for the hope that you have. But do this
with gentleness and respect, keeping a clear conscience . . ."*
1 PETER 3:15–16

It all comes down to hope. You were able to start Walking the Walk with me, and have kept doing so, because you had hope in your heart to begin with. You may have thought you were hopeless at first, but even then, at your lowest times, there was still hope in your heart. It was just dormant. Now it has burst into flower for all to see. Don't be afraid to show others your hope, to tell them that a bedrock of faith has been your foundation from the beginning. You shouldn't do this in a bragging way, but with gentleness and respect, so that they, too, can find the path that you've found.

Who out there needs to hear your good news? Who needs to know that they can do it, too? Hope is one of the most beautiful feelings anyone can have. Best of all, you can share yours and still have just as much as you started with.

↙ Activities ↝

Try any of these activities as a way to give what you've got.

- *Have a walking party at your house! Invite some coworkers or friends and introduce them to the joys of in-home walking. They'll thank you for the rest of their (healthy, happy) lives.*
- *If you have children at home, why not invite them to walk with you. Kids usually have a blast doing the steps and exercises! And if they see you walking with a smile on your face, they are going to associate physical activity and good health with happiness. You couldn't be giving them a better start!*
- *You don't have to get others to walk with you to make your walking contribute to their lives. Use your newfound energy and optimism to make an impression on a young person and change that person's life. Think of a specific thing you can do to get someone started on the path of healthy living, and do it this week.*

↙ Fit Facts ↝

Teen Sleep

The average teen needs nine hours of sleep a night, and usually gets it on weekends and in the summer. During the school week, however, the average teen gets only seven hours of sleep a night—not nearly enough. This shows up in poor performance, mood, and health. (Teens also perform better on afternoon tests than on morning tests.) Teens' biological clocks seem to be programmed for sleeping in, so let them, if you can. Encourage your school district to push back its start time and you'll have done a favor for all the kids in your town.

Getting Bigger

In 2004, 14 percent of American children between the ages of two and five were overweight. That's up from 10 percent in 2000. Overall, 17 percent of kids are overweight, while 66 percent of adults are.

Kids and Soda

Kids drink twice as much soda as water. The average teen pours 1.5 pounds of sugar down her throat each week in the form of soda. This is one of the big reasons 17 percent of kids are overweight and the incidence of diabetes is soaring among children. It's partly why more kids are breaking bones, due to more sugar and less calcium in their diets. And it's why, thanks to a deal the beverage companies have made with former president Bill Clinton, you won't see sugary sodas in schools much longer. By 2010, only diet sodas, bottled water, fruit juices, and milk will be allowed in school vending machines. That could cut hundreds of empty calories out of our children's daily diets and significantly improve their health. Next task: ridding schools of junk food.

Doing It for Them

Affirmation

"Every day I walk, I'm contributing not just to my own quality of life but to the quality of all the lives that touch mine."

Today's Walk

How Far? _____

Strength Training? _____

How'd It Go? _____

Notes

_____

_____

_____

DAY 29

Your Call to Service

Yesterday, we focused on the benefits of modeling good behavior—how the payback you receive from Walking the Walk spills over and encourages others, especially kids, to make healthy decisions also. But that's just one aspect of your deeper mission, which is a call to service that involves not just cleaning up your own act and serving as an example to others but devoting your life to others and to God.

This call to service can take a million different forms; anything counts that contributes to creating and sustaining a just, kind, faithful, healthy, thriving, and loving society. You get to pick all the ways that resonate most profoundly for you. But pick carefully, because you don't want to make your commitments out of a sense of duty, but because service and generosity are the most direct path to joy.

Some people mistakenly think of giving as a trade-off: If I do some nice things for other people, then God will do some nice things for me. But that's not the idea. The very act of doing things for other people *becomes* a blessing for yourself. The act is the reward. Once you change your perspective to one that values service and kindness above all things, you get the joy and fulfillment you crave simply by doing good.

You may hear people say, "Whatever you give, you shall receive ten-fold," or some other variation on "reaping what you sow." The idea is true, but that's not why you should give. It shouldn't be like investing in the stock market. You are putting yourself first if you think, Gee, if I do three favors for people, I'll get thirty back in the future! And if you are your main focus, neither thirty favors nor three hundred are going to bring you happiness. Your happiness is not the goal; it's the by-product of right living. If you dwell on yourself and what is wrong in your own life, you can always find something that is wrong or someone who has something that you don't.

When you genuinely embrace your call to service, with no calculations about what *you* will get out of it, then everything changes. The problems in your life that you thought were unsolvable suddenly disappear because, with your new focus on others, they aren't even problems anymore. You didn't "solve" them; you redefined them out of existence! Not being a millionaire, for example, is only a problem if you consider being a millionaire a prerequisite to happiness. By changing your value system, you can get the same sense of accomplishment and joy from serving a bowl of soup to someone who really needs it that a commodities trader gets from making his first million. In fact, if happiness surveys are to be believed, you'll probably get *more*. The things most likely to bring about happiness are connection to others, generosity, and a sense of deeper purpose in one's life.

Let's get back to the call to service. If everybody has a little bit of God in them, then whenever you serve others, you are serving God. That's an easy principle to keep in mind. How much of your life is about helping others? Can you do more? Remember that you do need to take care of yourself so that you will be able to make your contributions; that's what this thirty-day program is about. Now, with your energy and confidence surging from all that exercise and spiritual fire, see if you can channel it into helping create a world of excellence and integrity.

◡꙳ Having Faith ◠

See if you recognize yourself in any of these un-faith-full thought patterns. Today, try to switch your inner dialogue so that your mind walks the walk along with your body.

Un-Faith-Full Thoughts:

- ꙮ Nobody ever helped me get to where I am in life, so why should I help others?

- I'd like to do more volunteer work, but I just don't have the time. Things are so busy right now.
- Once I get rich, then I'll retire early and start giving my money away.

Walking the Walk:

"The changes I've made in my health through regular walking have improved my life so much and hardly cost me a cent. I wonder what other easy ways I can think of to improve the world around me?"

⌁ Walking for Other Reasons ~

"If you have any encouragement from being united with Christ, if any comfort from his love, if any fellowship with the Spirit, if any tenderness and compassion, then make my joy complete by being like-minded, having the same love, being one in spirit and purpose. Do nothing out of selfish ambition or vain conceit, but in humility consider others better than yourselves. Each of you should look not only to your own interests, but also to the interests of others."

PHILIPPIANS 2:1–4

Being the best at something is rarely a route to happiness. Sure, it feels better to win than to lose, but it's a lonely sort of satisfaction that comes from being at the top and defending your perch. Deep satisfaction comes from sharing with others, from understanding that we are all in this together and nobody is any better than anyone else. In fact, if you can "consider others better than yourself," as Paul says, then you take a huge step forward in achieving the joy that comes with working with one spirit and purpose for the benefit of all.

Remember, this does not mean that God is asking you to quit your job, join the clergy, and feed the poor every day. That's one way to further God's work, but there are countless others. Most jobs exist because there is a need for them. People need many, many different services. Finding your calling means not so much choosing a "virtuous" profession but, rather, choosing something you are good at and doing it to the best of your ability, with virtue, integrity, and class. Put your natural skills into the world and exercise them unselfishly, for the good of all. That's the route to bliss.

◡ Activities ◠

Try any of these activities as a way to orient yourself toward service to others.

- *Go hug somebody. That's the easiest activity in this entire book, and maybe the best! Why do we all hold back with our hugs? Because we worry we'll run out? Somebody out there needs your hug! Find them and make their day.*
- *Consider your daily occupation. Ask yourself if it meets these two criteria: 1. You enjoy it. 2. You feel good about the impact it has. If you answered no to either one of these, then ask yourself what is holding you back from finding a more gratifying calling. What changes could you make to start getting closer to that gratification?*
- *Think about the figures who made the biggest impact on your maturation. Envision their lives and motivations. What drove them, and how much of their life was devoted to others? Would they approve of your life today? If not, what changes could you make so that they would be proud of you all over again?*

◡ Fit Facts ◠

Are You in the Right Job?

Only 50 percent of Americans are satisfied with their jobs, down 10 percent from ten years ago. Fourteen percent of those earning more than fifty thousand dollars are "very satisfied," while 17 percent of those earning less than fifteen thousand are "very satisfied." Workers in the Middle Atlantic and Mountain states were the least satisfied, while those in the Southeast were the most satisfied. But what are the most telling statistics showing that way too many Americans are choosing their careers for the wrong reasons? Forty percent said they felt disconnected from their employers, 67 percent did not feel compelled by their company's goals and objectives, and 25 percent said they were just showing up for the paycheck. If any of these describe you, make a change while you still have time to enjoy it!

Diabetes Goes Global

We've heard a lot about the scourge of diabetes in the United States, but the 20 million people with the disease nationally pales compared to the 230 million around the world with diabetes, and the projected 350 million by 2025. In some countries, 20 percent of the population has diabetes. The problem is worst in Third World countries, and the culprits are familiar to us: more sedentary lifestyles and a diet too high in starches and sugars.

Fun in the Sun 101

Skin cancer is on the rise worldwide, and part of the reason is our misuse of sunscreen. Did you know that to get the full SPF rating listed on the package, you need to apply at least a *full ounce* of lotion? And you need to apply it at least fifteen minutes before going out in the sun, so it has time to form a barrier on your skin. Also, look for a sunscreen that blocks UVA and UVB rays, both of which cause cancer. And don't count on your beach pullover to do the job of sunscreen; a T-shirt has an SPF of only 10 at best. One of the best things you can do to protect your skin for life is to wear a wide-brimmed hat whenever you go outside. Some hats and clothes are now made with built-in SPF factors; they are worth a try!

Your Call to Service

Affirmation

"Today I will make somebody else's day!"

Today's Walk

How Far? _____

Strength Training? _____

How'd It Go? _____

Notes

_____

_____

_____

Walking in Love

When biologists assess the health of ecosystems, they have what they call "umbrella species." These are species, such as the grizzly bear, that range so widely and rely on so many different species and factors for their survival that if they are doing well, it means most of the other species under their "umbrella" must be doing well, too. It's almost impossible to stay aware of the health of every part of an ecosystem, so umbrella species serve as a shortcut.

The ecosystem that is you has its own umbrella species. It's called love. We've spent thirty days looking at some of the many ways to support a spiritually and physically fit life. You could go through them one by one and see how well you're doing in each, or you can use the shortcut: If love flows through your life and is an important part of your decisions and happiness, then you can be pretty sure your whole "ecosystem" is healthy.

By now, I hope you've connected two concepts in your mind: movement and love. Movement is life, and life is love. To keep living, you must keep moving ahead. You don't get attached to the past or to your current spot; you just keep getting better and more capable, keep achieving your next goal. Loving the adventure of it all and embracing the new you are the best ways to keep love strong in your life.

As you do this, don't make the mistake of thinking that embracing the new you means there was anything wrong with the old you. Movement and energy are what keep life vibrant, but you aren't leaving behind anything bad. Love the way you're headed and the place you came from equally. While it's important to achieve, to keep putting one foot in front of the other, you don't need to prove anything. You are not incomplete. You are already a whole and wholly lovable person. That's the lesson of God's love.

Think about how many of your actions are driven by a need to prove yourself somehow, either to yourself or to others. Then think about how often other people are trying to prove something to you by how they look, how much money they have, or how good they are at something. How different would life be if all these exchanges, which are driven by the fear of being found unacceptable somehow, were instead driven by mutual love. One of the great comforts Christians have when they meet is knowing that love for all mankind is a shared value. Knowing that, they can quickly move on to manifesting that love in the world.

Walking in love doesn't mean that you'll stop accomplishing anything and will just spend the rest of your life on the couch, basking in divine love and an inner sense of completeness. In fact, you'll do just the opposite. When you have nothing to prove and have no fears weighing you down, you discover that it is far more natural to interact with the world, expressing your love, than it is to stay isolated.

When you walk today, walk in love—love for yourself, for God, for all the people who make your life what it is, and for all the other people, too. You are complete, you have arrived, you are perfect in yourself. There is no better way to express love than to help other people discover the same truth.

⌣ Having Faith ∿

See if you recognize yourself in any of these un-faith-full thought patterns. Today, try to switch your inner dialogue so that your mind walks the walk along with your body.

Un-Faith-Full Thoughts:

ↄ My friends and family know that I love them. I don't need to tell them.

- I feel a lot of love in my heart, but if I show this to other people, they will make fun of me.
- There are some people worthy of my love, but a lot of others are mean-spirited and I just write them off.

Walking the Walk:
**"Love is God's essence, and I won't let others' fears
keep me from feeling that love and sharing it."**

⌁ Walking for Other Reasons ⌁

*". . . God is love. Whoever lives in love lives in God,
and God in him. In this way, love is made complete among
us so that we will have confidence on the day of judgment,
because in this world we are like him. There is no fear in love.
But perfect love drives out fear, because fear has to do with
punishment. The one who fears is not made perfect in love."*
1 John 4:16–18

What an amazing life it would be if we were able to keep love in our hearts at all times and never act out of fear! With true love and faithfulness, you never lose your way or get knocked off balance by someone else's actions. True love has its own honor code.

True love doesn't look for reciprocation.

True love doesn't judge (not even yourself).

True love doesn't show off.

True love doesn't cheat or lie.

True love doesn't offend or put down.

True love doesn't ignore.

True love doesn't get defensive.

True love has no fear.

True love doesn't mind losing.

True love helps everyone win.

⌣ Activities ⌣

Try any of these activities as a way to spread God's love.

- *Pretend someone asked you, "If you could pick one word to sum up what your life's about, what would that word be?" Choose your word. If that word was anything other than* love, *ask yourself why. What would change if, starting today, you did make love the focus of your life?*
- *No matter who you are, sometimes people are going to treat you badly. Follow Christ's example by making an effort to respond to hostility, ridicule, suspicion, judgment, and even indifference with love. How does this change the way you feel?*
- *The next time you meet a stranger, treat him or her as you would a loved family member. Make the same assumptions you would for siblings or cousins—that they like you, trust you, would go out of their way to help you, and would never do you wrong. Chances are that all these things are true anyway, so what do you have to lose?*

⌣ Fit Facts ⌣

Holding Hands

Researchers studying pain thresholds found that women who held their husbands' hands experienced less pain and stress from an electric shock than women who held either a stranger's hand or no one's hand. No surprise there; previous studies have found that happily married couples live longer than others, with better overall health and less sickness from colds and flu.

Love Loves Love

A major study at the University of Chicago found that people who had strong romantic relationships also had the highest feelings of altruistic love in general. Among married people, 40 percent scored in the highest ranking for altruistic love, while only 27 percent of divorced people and 20 percent of never-married people scored in the highest ranking. Religion is also an important support for altruism. Those who prayed daily were the most likely group to perform altruistic acts.

Pet Love

Fifty-eight percent of pet owners would skip work to take care of their sick pet, and 73 percent would gladly go into debt to keep their pets well. Now, that's altruism!

Walking in Love

Affirmation

"I love my life!"

Today's Walk

How Far? _____

Strength Training? _____

How'd It Go? _____

Notes

_____

_____

_____

A Witness for Fitness

Jennifer Antkowiak

Pittsburgh, Pennsylvania

When I met Leslie, I was about six months away from having my fifth baby—my fifth in less than nine years! I was back at work in a demanding full-time job as a television newscaster at KDKA-TV in Pittsburgh. Besides anchoring an evening newscast, I hosted a morning talk and information show called Pittsburgh Today Live. *I was looking to find a way to fit a fitness program into my busy lifestyle, but nothing seemed to work. I had a gym membership, but after being away from the kids all day, the last thing I wanted to do was something that would keep me away from them any longer.*

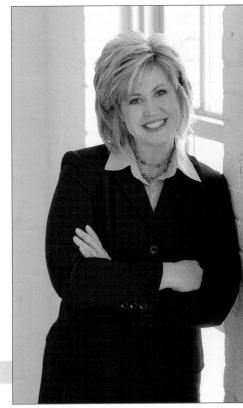

I saw an article in a magazine about a walking program you could do in your home. What is this crazy thing? I thought. I mentioned it to my producer, and she knew of Leslie Sansone, and knew that Leslie lived in New Castle, only an hour away from Pittsburgh. We arranged for Leslie to appear on our show. That one appearance turned into a regular monthly segment where Leslie would walk with us, motivate us, and give us our Walk Diet for the month.

I walked right along with our viewers, and lost seventeen pounds in six weeks! I loved Leslie's energy . . . loved the fact that the program was so easy to follow . . . loved that I could make it fit into my crazy schedule. (Many times, the kids would wake up and find me walking in our family room in my pajamas!)

I loved walking with Leslie so much, loved the

healthy message she's spreading to millions of people, that I walked right out of my seventeen-year television career to help her! Now I'm working with Leslie to spread the message to busy women, families, and children. We are working to produce healthy-lifestyle programming, including nutrition segments, for television and the Web to help people on their fitness journeys.

I feel so blessed to be in this position! The work is creative and energizing and I'm able to do it and still have plenty of time with my family. I've also been able to build regular exercise into my schedule, and now I've lost thirty pounds with Leslie's programs!

I hope other busy moms will connect with me, and see that if I can do it, they can, too . . . because they really can. I'm sure of it.

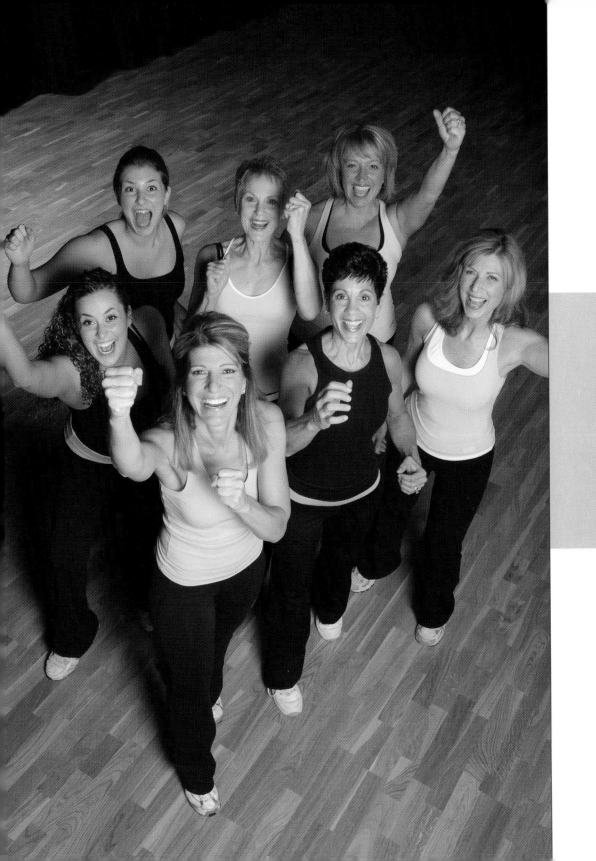

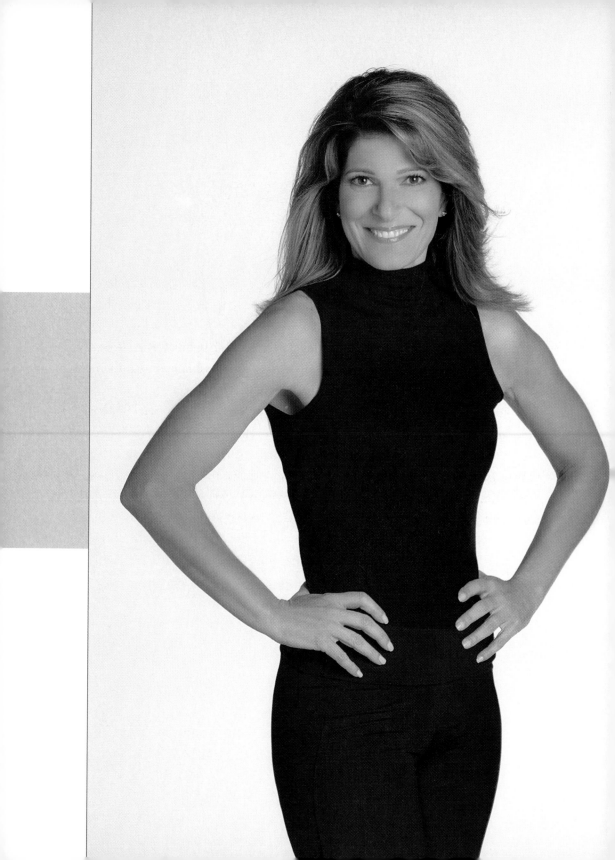

Thirty Days Down,
One Lifetime to Go!

Congratulations! You have delivered on your promise. For thirty days, you've made an impressive commitment, and your spirit is flourishing because of it. I hope my program has been helpful to you, but—as you may have discovered—you don't owe your success to this book or to me. It was all you. Your success came from within, and that successful spirit was there all along, waiting for an opportunity to bloom.

Now, how do you keep your spirit blooming for the rest of your life? By avoiding the activities or thought patterns that caused it to go dormant in the first place. If you have picked up useful habits in this book that help you stay fit physically and mentally, that help you achieve less body, more soul, then by all means keep doing them. If other activities were not useful, then you get to leave them behind. It's your choice! The only rule is to stay true to your spirit.

When you reach a point where you're ready to share your success with the world, *please* let me hear from you! Go to www.LeslieSansone.com and tell me all about it. I love to let others know the good news! When we walk hand in hand with God, all things are possible! "A closer walk with thee" is my prayer for you and for me. Your body is God's temple; may He dwell in you always. Now, *go forth and walk!*

All My Blessings,

Leslie Sansone

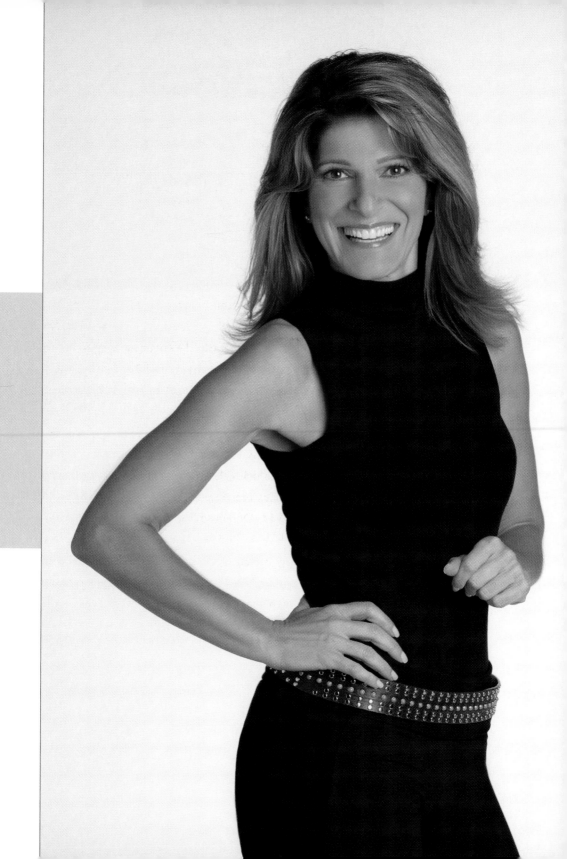

Appendix

Seven-Day "Jump Start" Weight-Loss Plan

We all know that to lose serious weight we need to exercise daily *and* eat healthy meals. Some people enjoy creating their own meal plans; others like to have meal plans they can follow. If you are one of those who would rather put your energy into something other than meal planning, have I got a treat for you! It's the Seven-Day "Jump Start" Weight-Loss Plan. I call it the "Jump Start" plan because it will put you *well* down the road to fitness before you even realize you've begun!

Here's all you do. Each day, read a chapter in this book for inspiration, then follow the supersimple meal plans found here. Each meal is approximately five hundred to six hundred calories, keeping you in a range of fifteen hundred to eighteen hundred calories per day. Then, do all three miles as shown on the *Walking the Walk* DVD. Depending on your fitness level and intensity, you will burn around four hundred calories—almost an entire meal! Give yourself six days (on the seventh, we rest) and you will shake up your body, mind, and spirit like never before! The following week, you can adjust your walking and eating to fit your lifestyle goals, or you can begin your "jump start" week all over again if you want to keep your weight loss at a fever pitch!

Day 1

Breakfast

 Drink a glass of water before eating!

Bowl of oatmeal (use old-fashioned oats, not instant oatmeal) with skim milk and just 1 teaspoon of brown sugar or maple syrup
Hard-boiled egg
Coffee or tea

Lunch

 Drink a glass of water before eating!

½ turkey and cheese sandwich
1 cup low-fat yogurt—add berries of your choice
Optional nutrient boost: Sprinkle flaxseed on the yogurt.

Dinner

 Drink a glass of water before eating!

Seared or grilled fish (healthiest choice: salmon)
Salad of mixed greens with light dressing
Green tea

Day 2

Breakfast

 Drink a glass of water before eating!

Bowl of GOLEAN Crunch! cereal by Kashi (or your favorite whole-grain cereal) with skim milk
Natural peanut butter (no sugar added) on a banana
Coffee or tea

*"With Leslie's help,
I'm halfway to my goal.
Praise God!"*

LESLIE ANDERSON

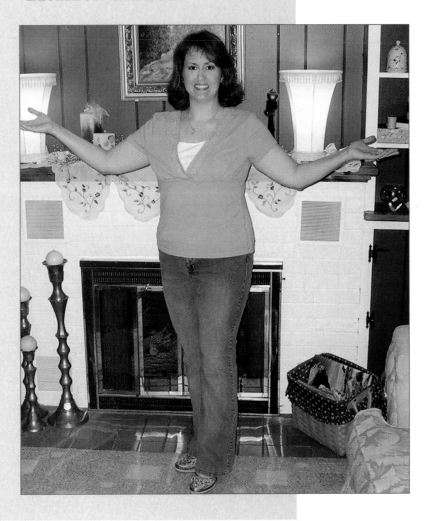

Lunch

 Drink a glass of water before eating!

1 cup chicken soup (clear broth, not creamy)
½ grilled cheese sandwich
Apple

Dinner

 Drink a glass of water before eating!

1 cup bow-tie pasta with broccoli
Grilled chicken breast, seasoned with garlic, olive oil, salt, and pepper
Green tea

Day 3

Breakfast

 Drink a glass of water before eating!

2 scrambled eggs (spray pan lightly with cooking spray)
2 pieces whole-grain toast with a pat of butter
Coffee or tea

Lunch

 Drink a glass of water before eating!

1 4-ounce can of tuna (drained)
Whole-grain crackers (150-calorie portion)
Cottage Doubles (these are individual portions of cottage cheese with fruit, sold everywhere)
Pear

"I am totally blind, but with Leslie I am able to follow every step and back kick without fail. If not for Leslie, I would not be able to do such a workout in my own home. Leslie has truly been the answer to my prayers. In five months, I have lost thirty-nine pounds, my cholesterol has dropped, and my doctor cut my blood-pressure medication in half."

JENNY PIPER

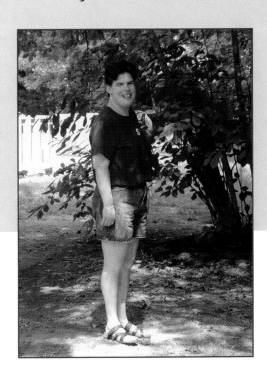

Dinner

 Drink a glass of water before eating!

Steak (1 portion is the size and thickness of the palm of your hand)
Baked potato with a pat of butter
Salad of mixed greens with light dressing
Green tea

Day 4

Breakfast

 Drink a glass of water before eating!

2 whole-grain pancakes topped with a teaspoon of natural peanut butter and
maple syrup (you earned a treat for walking all those miles!)
Coffee or tea

Lunch

 Drink a glass of water before eating!

Whole-grain chips (200-calorie portion)
Salsa
1 cup low-fat yogurt
1 cup berries of your choice

Dinner

 Drink a glass of water before eating!

Grilled white fish (cod, flounder, sea bass, catfish, etc.), seasoned with olive
oil, garlic, lemon, salt, and fresh herbs of your choice
Mixed grilled vegetables, seasoned the same as the fish
Green tea

Day 5

Breakfast

 Drink a glass of water before eating!

Bowl of whole-grain cereal with skim milk
1 whole-grain English muffin with peanut butter or jam
Coffee or tea

Lunch

 Drink a glass of water before eating!

1 4-ounce can of sardines packed in olive oil (or tuna if you don't like
   sardines)
Whole-grain crackers (200-calorie portion)
Apple

Dinner

 Drink a glass of water before eating!

Chicken breast (prepared any way you desire)
1 cup brown rice
Fresh spinach salad with light dressing
Green tea

Day 6

Breakfast

 Drink a glass of water before eating!

Bowl of oatmeal (old-fashioned, not instant) with skim milk and just 1
   teaspoon of brown sugar or maple syrup

"I use Leslie's videos for my missionary work in Africa. Thank you so much and have a good walking day!"

ANNIE BELLAVITI

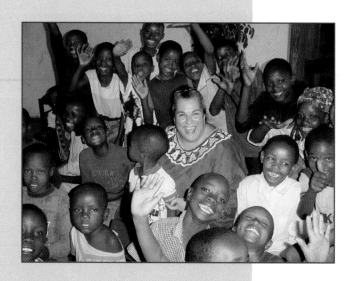

Hard-boiled egg
Coffee or tea

Lunch

 Drink a glass of water before eating!

1 cup of soup (clear broth, not creamy)
½ tuna sandwich
1 handful walnuts
Orange

Dinner

 Drink a glass of water before eating!

Whole-wheat pasta with marinara sauce
Salad of mixed greens with light dressing
Green tea

Day 7

Rest! Eat what you want. Drink what you want. Do what you want. You have
earned this special day!

Some of My Favorite Superfoods!

☺ Oatmeal   ☺ Eggs or Egg Whites
☺ Salmon / Sardines   ☺ Flaxseed
☺ Olive Oil (extra virgin) ☺ Yogurt
☺ Broccoli / Spinach   ☺ Walnuts
☺ Garlic   ☺ Whole-Grain Breads and Pastas
☺ Berries   ☺ Green Tea

Throughout the week, check the smiley face next to any of these foods
that you eat. If your weekly diet includes most of these supernutritious foods,
then you know you are really Walking the Walk! Bravo!

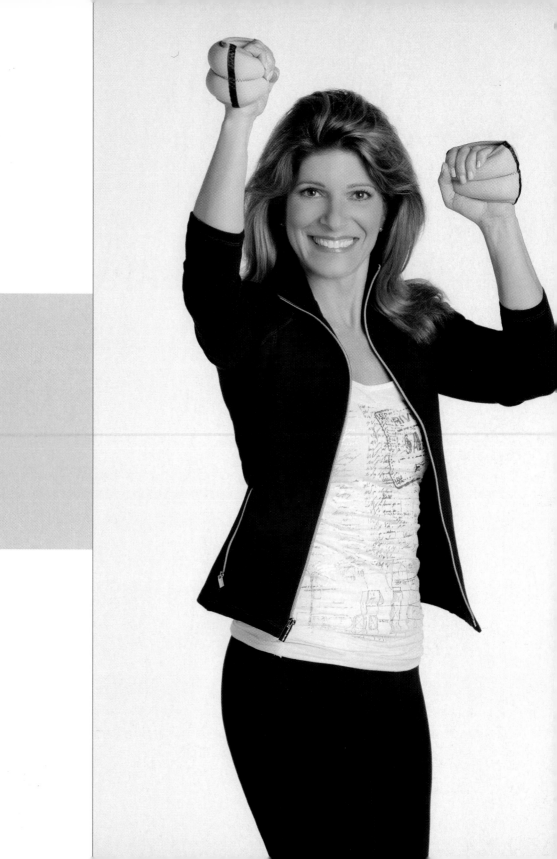